Nursing - New Insights for Clinical Care

Edited by Victor Chaban

Published in London, United Kingdom

Nursing - New Insights for Clinical Care
http://dx.doi.org/10.5772/intechopen.98014
Edited by Victor Chaban

Contributors
Dilar Costa, Joana Matias, Filipa Aguiar, Amr Salem, Onyinye Allen Nwachukwu, Sabahat Zafar, Luis Yovera Leyva, Oana Velicu-Scraba, Venkata Sirisha Gurram, Sachi Sri Kantha, Motohiro Sano, Tomoko Majima, Parisa Bozorgzad, Nazri Nordin, Princess Busisiwe Siphiwe Mbatha, Maged Shendy, Delia Marinceu, Hanadi Dakhilallah, Mohua Roy, Amar Siddique, Adelaide Maria Ansah Ofei, Yennutin Paarima, Theresa Barnes

First published in London, United Kingdom, 2023 by IntechOpen
IntechOpen is the global imprint of INTECHOPEN LIMITED, registered in England and Wales, registration number: 11086078, 5 Princes Gate Court, London, SW7 2QJ, United Kingdom

British Library Cataloguing-in-Publication Data
A catalogue record for this book is available from the British Library

Additional hard and PDF copies can be obtained from orders@intechopen.com

Nursing - New Insights for Clinical Care
Edited by Victor Chaban
p. cm.
Print ISBN 978-1-80355-516-4
Online ISBN 978-1-80355-517-1
eBook (PDF) ISBN 978-1-80355-518-8

Meet the editor

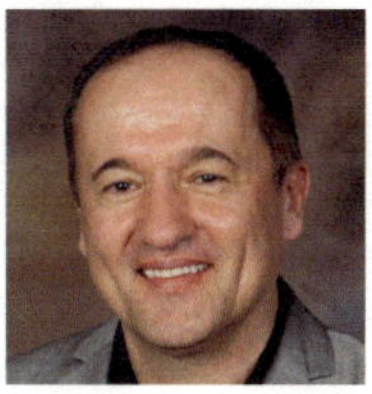

Dr. Victor V. Chaban is a Chairman of the Department of Biomedical Science Education and Professor of Medicine with a dual appointment at the Charles R. Drew University of Medicine and Science (CDU) and the University of California Los Angeles (UCLA). Dr. Chaban completed his post-doctoral training in neuroscience at UCLA and his graduate studies in clinical research at CDU. He has served on the US National Institute of Health and several international study sections and holds US patents. Dr. Chaban is Editor in Chief for the *International Journal of Research* in Nursing and serves on several editorial boards. He is the author of four books. His new book, *Calcium Signaling and Nervous System* was published by Nova Medicine and Health, New York in 2020.

Contents

Preface

This book provides a comprehensive and up-to-date overview of current nursing practice and clinical interventions. The authors are a group of international experts with a focus on the clinical aspects upon which the practice components of nursing care are based. We hope that many of the technological and therapeutic advances described will allow nurses and other healthcare professionals to use best practices to improve healthcare outcomes in different categories of patients. *Nursing - New Insights* for Clinical Care, however, does not aim to provide a compendium of recent advances in nursing care but rather to focus on current experiences in health care delivery. Today, understanding and meeting patient concerns is as important as performing therapeutic interventions, and information regarding the best approaches in healthcare delivery has increased significantly. Paradoxically, proposed therapeutic interventions are sometimes complicated by contradictory data, due to different methodological approaches to their collection. Evidence-based practice and guidelines to improve the efficiency of clinical interventions are therefore as important for the profession as for the public.

I wish to express my sincere thanks to all who have contributed to this book by describing the role of nurses in the treatment of different acute and/or chronic diseases, their etiology, pathogenesis, clinical outcomes, and symptomatic presentation. Each chapter focuses on specific nursing interventions due to advances in international healthcare. Motohiro Sano and Tomoko Majima from Japan describe a home-based heart failure nursing intervention supporting self-management and independent living. Dilar Costa, Joana Matias and Filipa Aguiar from Portugal show the importance of the dialogue between renal transplant patients' educational needs and the knowledge transmitted by nurses. Shendy Majed from the UK discusses the role of nursing in urogynecology. Adelaide Maria Ansah Ofei, Yennuten Paarima and Theresa Barnes from Ghana explore strategic leadership in nursing. Amr Salem from the UK describes the management of obstetric and intrapartum emergencies. Parisa Bozorgzad from Iran studies the cultural safety of hospitalized patients. Sachi Sri Kantha from Japan presents recent findings on somnambulism. Mbatha Princess Busisive Siphive from South Africa demonstrates the use of the Lautenbach irrigation system in clinical practice. Nazri Nordin from Malaysia describes an advanced nursing approach to palliative care.

Today's nurses collaborate with interdisciplinary teams throughout care settings and have a significant effect on specific groups of patients, particularly in the prevention of adverse events or comorbidity of symptoms. While it is very difficult to provide an overview of all aspects of nursing, we hope that this book will be a valuable resource not only for nurses but for other clinicians, students and patients seeking insights into new therapies and clinical practices.

Victor Chaban, Ph.D., MS
Professor and Chairman,
Department of Biomedical Science Education,
Charles R. Drew University of Medicine and Science,
Los Angeles, CA, USA

Professor,
Department of Medicine,
University of California,
Los Angeles, CA, USA

Chapter 1

A Home-Based Heart Failure Nursing Intervention Supporting Self-Management and Lives

Motohiro Sano and Tomoko Majima

Abstract

In the era of a super-aged society, along with the rapid development of medical techniques to treat cardiovascular disease, there are an increasing number of aged patients with heart failure (HF). To cope with this near pandemic, coordinated-HF management combining hospital-based optimal therapy and home-based care is required. Accordingly, the concept of "living with HF" is advocated and is widely accepted as a key to improve patients' quality of life as well as prognosis. To achieve it, home visiting nursing services are essential. But these services have some difficulties. This chapter shows the importance of promoting self-management for patients with heart failure and intervention strategies in the home care setting.

Keywords: heart failure, self-management, re-hospitalization, home-based intervention, home visiting nursing

1. Introduction

HF is the quintessential cardiovascular syndrome of aging that results from age-related cardiovascular conditions and age-associated changes in cardiovascular structure and function. The prevalence of HF among approximately 1–2% of the adult population in developed countries, rising to ≧10% among those over 70 years of age and the most common reason for hospitalization in older adults. Usually, as studies only include diagnosed HF cases, the true prevalence is likely to be higher [1, 2]. Although some progress has been made in reducing mortality in patients with HF, rates of rehospitalization continue to rise and approach 40–50% within 1 year after discharge [3, 4]. To reduce mortality and rehospitalization rate, it is widely recognized that, in addition to optimizing medical and device therapies for HF, attention should also be given to how HF care is delivered. Several position papers that cover non-pharmacological management, discharge planning, and standards for delivering HF care.

Appropriate self-management by patients with HF plays an important role in the prevention of HF decompensation and improvement of survival and quality of life (QOL) [5]. A literature review stated that most HF treatment figure on self-management intervention and focus on self-management strategies, such as to become more informed about their illness and be actively engaged in their own care, which is necessary to improve the impact of self-management on long-term heart failure outcomes [6]. Therefore, nurses should play a key role in improving self-management by comprehensive patient assessment, patient-centered goal setting, evaluation of outcomes, encouraging health promotion, and self-management education. In addition, self-management for patients with HF support should be a part of routine health care, and effective strategies still need to be embedded into routine care. However, a study that surveyed the knowledge of community nurses revealed that they had a basic understanding of HF but scored poorly on weight assessment, blood pressure management, and reporting to physicians of dizziness [7]. This chapter focuses on self-management and lifestyle advice for patients with HF to prevent exacerbation and rehospitalization in the home setting.

2. Types of HF

Traditionally, HF has been divided into three phenotypes based on the measurement of left ventricular ejection fraction (LVEF). Reduced LVEF is defined as ≦40%, and left ventricular systolic dysfunction. This is designated as heart failure with reduced ejection fraction (HFrEF). Mildly reduced LVEF is defined as between 41% and 49%. Clinical features and prognosis have not yet been fully characterized. This is designated as heart failure with mildly reduced ejection fraction (HFmrEF). Those with symptoms and signs of HF, with evidence of structural and/or functional cardiac abnormalities and/or raised natriuretic peptides (NPs), and with an LVEF ≥ 50%, have heart failure with preserved ejection fraction (HFpEF). No effective treatments have been established. The simplest terminology used to describe the severity of HF is the New York Heart Association (NYHA) functional classification.

The etiology of HF varies according to geography. In western countries and developed countries, coronary artery disease and hypertension are predominant factors. With regard to ischemic etiology, HFmrEF resembles HFrEF, with a higher frequency of underlying CAD compared to those with HFpEF. **Table 1** shows the definition of HF based on LVEF [1].

The simplest terminology used to describe the severity of HF is the New York Heart Association (NYHA) functional classification. The NYHA functional classification was developed by the New York Heart Association as a system to classify patients with heart diseases according to the severity of symptoms resulting from physical

Type		**HFrEF**	**HFmrEF**	**HFpEF**
Criteria	1	Symptoms ± signs	Symptoms ± signs	Symptoms ± signs
	2	LVEF ≦ 40%	LVEF 41–49%	LVEF ≧ 50%
	3	Mainly contractile insufficiency. Many current studies include her cases of decreased LVEF under standard heart failure treatment as HFrEF	The presence of elevated natriuretic peptides and other structural heart diseases	Objective evidence of cardiac structural and/or functional abnormalities consistent with the presence of LV diastolic dysfunction/ raised LV filling pressures, including raised natriuretic peptides

HF, heart failure; LV, left ventricular; LVEF, left ventricular ejection fraction.

Table 1.
Definition of HF with reduced ejection fraction, mildly reduced ejection fraction, and preserved ejection fraction.

activity and has been used in the severity classification of HF. NYHA class II patients were further classified into those with slight limitation of physical activity (IIs) and those with moderate limitation of physical activity (IIm).

NYHA I is "No limitation of physical activity. Ordinary physical activity does not cause severe fatigue, palpitations, dyspnea or angina."

NYHA II is "Slight or moderate limitation of physical activity. Comfortable at rest, but ordinary physical activity causes fatigue, palpitations, dyspnea or angina."

NYHA III is "Marked limitation of physical activity. Comfortable at rest, but less than ordinary activity causes fatigue, palpitations, dyspnea or angina."

NYHA IV is "Unable to carry on any physical activity without symptoms of HF, or symptoms of HF and angina at rest. Even slight activity worsens symptoms."

3. Risk factors of exacerbation of HF

HF can be prevented from developing, exacerbating, or recurring by various interventions, such as appropriate treatment and medication for risk factors for heart failure, in addition to lifestyle-related management such as diet and exercise. Smoking is a risk factor for cardiovascular disease, and smoking cessation is strongly recommended for smokers because quitting reduces the mortality rate and readmission rate for cardiovascular disease, including HF [8]. Obesity and diabetes are associated with the development of HF, and insulin resistance-based diabetes and metabolic syndrome are both major risk factors for cardiovascular disease and are commonly used in weight loss and exercise therapy. In addition to improving lifestyle habits, comprehensive risk management through comprehensive treatment is required [9]. To prevent the exacerbation of HF, nurses need to understand risk factors and prevention strategies. **Table 2** shows risk factors of exacerbation of HF.

Risk factors	Prevention strategies
Sedentary habit	Regular physical activity
Obesity	Physical activity and healthy diet
Cigarette smoking	Smoking cessation
Excessive alcohol	No/light alcohol intake is beneficial
Influenza	Influenza vaccination
Hypertension	Lifestyle changes, antihypertensive therapy
Dyslipidemia	Healthy diet, statins
Diabetes mellitus	Physical activity and healthy diet, SGLT2 inhibitors
Microbes	Early diagnosis, specific antimicrobial therapy for either prevention and/or treatment
CAD	Lifestyle changes, statin therapy
Chest radiation	Cardiac function and side effect monitoring, dose adaptation
Cardiotoxic drugs	Cardiac function and side effect monitoring, dose adaptation, change of chemotherapy

CAD, coronary artery disease; SGLT2, sodium-glucose co-transporter 2.

Table 2.
Risk factors of exacerbation of HF.

4. Importance of self-management for patients with HF

HF is one of the most common causes of hospital admissions and readmissions. A recent review revealed that nurse-led hospital-to-home transitional care interventions reduced the risk of all-cause mortality and heart failure-related hospitalizations, and improved health-related quality of life (HRQOL) and heart failure knowledge compared to usual care. The narrative summary of evidence for self-care behaviors showed positive intervention effects [10, 11]. Generally, nurse-led hospital-to-home transitional care interventions may play a beneficial role in decreasing mortality and improving HRQOL and self-care behaviors for patients with HF. Therefore, self-management is the cornerstone of HF management. Self-management comprises adherence to behaviors, such as maintaining a low sodium diet and medication regimen, as well as symptom monitoring to maintain physiological stability and response to symptoms when they occur [12]. However, there are some concerns. First, previous studies have different contents and modes of intervention, evaluation tools, and there is a publication bias in the outcome of quality of life, which might lead to selection bias, detection bias, and attention bias. Second, due to the diverse durations of interventions and length of follow-up, these factors may affect the long-term effects of self-management interventions. As stated above, further considerations are needed to show the optimal self-management interventions in patients with HF.

5. Processes of self-management and restructuring own lifestyles

To promote self-management for patients with HF and support their lives, nurses need to understand patients' perspectives. Sano et al. described the process of self-management among elderly patients with HF who had avoided re-hospitalization for over 2 years [13]. They identified three sub-concepts and one core-concept. **Table 3** shows core-concept and three sub-concepts of self-management of patients with HF [13].

Core-concept	
Balance between preventing decompensation and preferences	Begin new exercise or hobby within capabilities Adjust physical activity to reduce heart failure symptoms Modify diet to prevent decompensation. Tell friends and acquaintances about their own illness to avoid overeating or overwork. Choose how to modify their old lifestyle Make personal choices on how to avoid stress. Manage CHF without decompensation
Sub-concepts	
Perception of HF	Sudden development of heart failure symptoms. Cognition that heart failure contributes to uncomfortable feeling or cough, etc. Understanding of causes of heart failure from rehospitalization experience
Encountering a new situation	Understanding that heart failure can be caused by lifestyle Desire not to repeat rehospitalization or necessity for early consultation Daily activity evokes heart failure symptoms
Life coordination for HF	Thinking about lifestyle modification to avoid the discomfort associated with heart failure and additional treatment Limit activities to reduce heart strain Maintain a job or hobby to live meaningfully

Table 3.
Core-concept and sub-concepts.

DOI: http://dx.doi.org/10.5772/intechopen.102509

The sub-concepts were perception of heart failure, encountering a new situation, and life coordination for heart failure. The sub-concepts yielded a single core-concept—balance between preventing decompensation and preferences. Patients with HF experience each sub-concept in no particular order and acquire a lifestyle tailored to the condition of HF. Then, when the state of HF becomes stable, not only actions for preventing the worsening of HF but also their own values and preferences are taken in, and the balance between them is maintained. A conceptual model was developed to illustrate the interactive relationships among the sub-concepts and the core-concept (**Figure 1**). **Figure 1** shows a conceptual framework of self-management among patients with HF [13].

5.1 Perception of HF

This sub-concept means that patients with HF experienced the onset of HF by sudden dyspnea and abnormal changes in their bodies. As a result of seeking medical care, they subsequently learned that their abnormal changes were symptoms of HF. Sources of HF information included inpatient and outpatient settings, from medical staff and laypeople, they encountered in daily life. After hospitalization, patients with HF understand that the onset of HF and deterioration of symptoms was related to several factors, such as living habits, work and overwork, fluid retention, excessive salt intake, and untreated high blood pressure.

5.2 Encountering a new situation

This sub-concept means that once the patients with HF understood how HF was related to their lifestyle, they noticed how the hospital environment was different from their own life at home in terms of activity, reducing salt intake, and management of blood pressure. They began confronting the reality that simple acts, like putting on their socks or cutting their nails, would become more difficult after hospitalization.

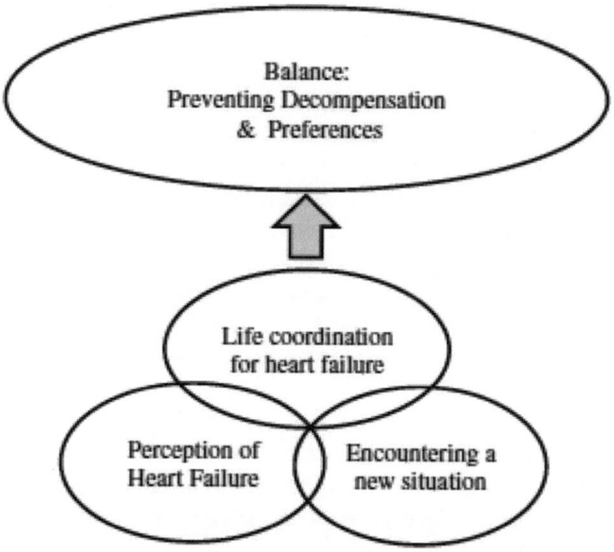

Figure 1.
Conceptual framework.

5.3 Life coordination

This sub-concept means that patients with HF reported that they did not want to experience that painful experience again. They believed that it had been a bad decision to just endure the pain and accept the abnormal physical changes as their condition became more severe. At the same time, they began to look back on their lifestyle selections; these led to behavioral modifications to avoid both painful experience and re-hospitalization. They understand that they could not continue living as they had before hospitalization; they could not avoid re-hospitalization if they did not change their lifestyle.

They also reported limiting their work. They began to adapt their lifestyle to one compatible with HF by limiting activities they had previously engaged in. Meanwhile, they were determined to continue living a worthwhile and energetic life.

5.4 Balance between preventing decompensation and preferences

This core-concept means that patients with HF try to maintain their agelong preferences to give their life a purpose, such as by maintaining long-term friendships and continuing to engage in interests. Instead of limiting all their activities, they stop engaging in activities that they learn would be bad for their heart and choose to continue those activities not be harmful.

They seek medical guidance to determine which activities were considered good for the heart or feasible within the scope of their limited lifestyle. They begin to reassemble their life into ones that do not put a strain on the heart while making up for lost parts of their life as a result of HF. They describe taking walks, singing a song, and engaging in new physical activities or hobbies within their realm of possibility. They determine which activities caused symptoms to appear and how far they could push themselves even if these were vacation activities or when invited by acquaintances. They make an effort to exercise at their own pace and master how to regulate their amount of exercise so as to avoid placing strain on the heart and causing symptoms.

They also utilize the knowledge they have acquired on limiting alcohol consumption and on excessive fluid and salt intake, which are related to water retention and edema. In doing so, they can prevent exacerbating their HF by modifying their diet. Nonetheless, they are faced with many situations that are difficult to avoid, such as opportunities to go drinking or eating out with others. In these situations, they make an effort to mitigate factors that would exacerbate their HF by avoiding overeating and overexertion, and by informing the people around them of their limits in advance. This allows patients to maintain their work and harmonious social lives while avoiding a diet that might lead to the exacerbation of HF.

Although they are aware of the need to modify their lifestyle, they believe that stress is worse and that it would be better to reduce stress by eating what they liked. Thus, they believe in prioritizing values over exacerbating their condition and giving priority to their preferences to avoid stress instead of respecting their limitations. They acknowledge having chosen to avoid stress over causing HF symptoms and pain. These thoughts, actions, and lifestyle choices demonstrate the complexly of symptom management in HF even when patients want to avoid exacerbating their condition. Apparently, they accept some deterioration because they want to act on their preferences and avoid the stress of compliance.

In summary, nurses need to recognize and value patients' views and experiences to support their self-care management.

6. Assessments of patients with HF for promoting self-management and supporting their lives

The self-management process is a process of living life such that symptoms do not worsen while balancing good choices and preferences. By trial and error, the patients with HF try to find the limits of physical capacity and dietary choices that would lead to the worsening of symptoms, while also trying to maintain quality of life to the extent possible [13]. Based on the process of self-management of patients with HF, it is possible to guide the assessment viewpoints to support self-management and their lives. It is important to understand the components of self-management. Components of self-management are "Experience and knowledge about HF," "Self-monitoring and Early perception," and "Life coordination for HF and to live meaningfully." The examples of the assessment viewpoints are shown below.

6.1 Experience and knowledge about HF

Acquisition and experience of knowledge about HF strongly contribute to the improvement of self-care skills, and lack of knowledge may decrease adherence and be a barrier to starting self-care behavior [12, 14]. In addition, patients with HF who understand and recognize the advice of medical professionals benefit the preventing worsening symptoms and readmission that can tend to have good adherence and perform self-care behavior [15]. In the process of self-management, knowledge and understanding of heart failure affect the entire self-management process and need to be continually confirmed even after moving from hospital to home. Assessment viewpoints include—(1) cognition that HF, (2) understanding of causes of HF (**Table 4**).

Assessment viewpoint	Example
Experience of the onset of HF, exacerbation, and hospitalization	How does the patient recognize the symptoms of heart failure?
	How does the patient perceive the symptoms of exacerbation of heart failure? (e.g. lower limb edema, shortness of breath, reduction of urine output, nocturnal cough, etc.)
Understanding causes of HF	Does the patient understand the behaviors/actions that lead to the exacerbation of heart failure? (e.g. inadequate physical activities, long haul travel, overactive, etc.)
	Does the patient understand the lifestyles that lead to the exacerbation of HF? (e.g. excessive alcohol and/or fluid and/or salt intake, smoking)

Table 4.
Assessment of experience and knowledge about HF.

6.2 Self-monitoring and early perception

It is said that less than half of the patients with HF regularly perform self-monitoring, such as measuring weight and confirming the degree of edema. The receiving treatment tends to be delayed due to the disagreement between the present HF symptoms and the patient's perception, but utilizing past knowledge and experience and receiving high-quality social support, it is possible to respond appropriately and early to the symptoms [16]. Symptom monitoring behavior is also a predictor of appropriate self-care management,

Assessment viewpoint	Example
Self-monitoring behaviors	Does the patient regularly measure his/her own weight and blood pressure?
	Does the patient regularly check the symptoms of HF? (e.g. lower limb edema, shortness of breath, reduction of urine output, nocturnal cough, etc.)
Self-monitoring circumstance	Does the patient has a sphygmomanometer and scale?
	Does the patient has a habit of maintaining track of his/her own conditions?
	Has the patient devised a way to remember the measurement and tracking?

Table 5.
Assessment of self-monitoring abilities.

and regular symptom monitoring for appropriate self-management practice is recommended [17]. To maintain and promote self-monitoring in patients with HF, we need to support patients with HF by performing daily monitoring, integrating knowledge, and past experiences regarding HF to determine how to evaluate their own conditions and take actions. **Table 5** shows the viewpoint of assessment of self-monitoring abilities.

6.3 Life coordination for HF and living meaningfully

In the stable period, excessive rest causes a decrease in exercise capacity and exacerbates fatigue and dyspnea during exertion, so moderate exercise increases exercise capacity, and it has been clarified that it leads to improvement of symptoms and improvement of QOL [5]. Appropriate exercise tolerance, evaluation of activities of daily living, and correction of physical activity and living behavior in consideration of physical function and living environment for each heart failure patient are required. **Table 6** shows the viewpoint of assessment of lifestyle and life circumstance.

6.4 Evaluation of exercise tolerance

Specific activity scale (SAS) specifies the metabolic equivalents (METs) for each physical activity, and it is possible to estimate the physical activity level from the

Assessment viewpoint	Example
Lifestyle and values	What are the long-standing hobbies and/or tastes?
	What about housework?
	What about regular exercise? (e.g. frequency, intensity, times, etc.)
	What about social activities and/or neighborhood relationships?
	Scheduled long-haul travel?
Life circumstance	Bedroom location (1st floor or 2nd floor? Using stairs?)
	How about installing bedding and handrails?
	Type and amount of seasoning
	What is the transportation for shopping and going out?
	Is there a steep slope in the neighborhood?

Table 6.
Assessment of lifestyle and life circumstance.

Ask questions about the following items and ask them to answer either "yes" or "no." The amount of exercise (METs) of the item for which the answer "no" appears for the first time is used as an index of the minimum amount of exercise in which symptoms appear		
Have a good sleeping	1MET	NYHA IV
Feel better when lay on the bed	1MET	
Eat something and wash face by yourself	1.6METs	
Could go to the toilet by yourself	2METs	NYHA III
Could change clothing by yourself	2METs	
Could prepare food and clean room	2-3METs	
Could prepare the bed by yourself	2-3METs	
Could clean the floor	3-4METs	
Could take shower by yourself	3-4METs	
Could walk 100-200 m on the ground as normal people	3-4METs	
Could clean the grass in the garden	4METs	
Could take a bath by yourself	4-5METs	NYHA II
Could go upstairs as a normal people	5-6METs	
Could do some light farm working	5-7METs	
Could walk fast on the ground	6-7METs	
Could play tennis	6-7METs	
Could do jogging (8 km/h) 300–400 m	7-8METs	NYHA I
Could do swimming	7-8METs	
Could skip rope	8METs	

Table 7.
SAS, METs, and the NYHA classification.

questionnaire [18]. METs are often used in clinical practice as a simple indicator of exercise intensity. NYHA classification is classified according to the degree of restriction of daily activities, and this classification is widely used for heart disease, especially in the stable period of HF. Its usefulness is high, and many reports have been made regarding its association with exercise tolerance and prognosis. The NYHA classification is simple and useful, but the content of the activity that is the basis of judgment is not clear, so SAS was developed to supplement it. SAS has tested the reproducibility and validity of the NYHA classification and METs. It is said to be more closely related to exercise tolerance and prognosis than the NYHA classification [19]. Physical activity that triggers the onset of HF symptoms is quantified by METs. **Table 7** shows the correspondence table between SAS, METs and NYHA classification [19].

7. Conclusions

HF is a severe public health problem all over the world. Adequate patient self-management is essential in the effective management of HF. Patients with HF who report more effective self-management have better QOL, lower readmission rates, and reduced mortality.

This chapter gives an overview of the current situation of patients with HF and self-management and shows the viewpoint of promoting self-management and supporting lifestyle. Supporting patient's life in the home setting, it is necessary to focus on their lifestyle, circumstance, and values before educational interventions. We believe that this chapter can be used not only for nurses in the home setting but also nurses in hospital settings who are involved with patients with HF at the time of discharge support.

Conflict of interest

The authors declares no conflict of interest.

Author details

Motohiro Sano* and Tomoko Majima
Graduate School of Nursing, Chiba University, Chiba City, Japan

*Address all correspondence to: sano-m@chiba-u.jp

References

[1] McDonagh TA, Metra M, Adamo M, Gardner RS, Baumbach A, Böhm M, et al. 2021 ESC guidelines for the diagnosis and treatment of acute and chronic heart failure. European Heart Journal. 2021;**42**(36):3599-3726

[2] Dharmarajan K, Rich MW. Epidemiology, pathophysiology, and prognosis of heart failure in older adults. Heart Failure Clinics. 2017;**13**(3):417-426

[3] Crespo-Leiro MG, Anker SD, Maggioni AP, Coats AJ, Filippatos G, Ruschitzka F, et al. European Society of Cardiology Heart Failure Long-Term Registry (ESC-HF-LT): 1-year follow-up outcomes and differences across regions. European Journal of Heart Failure. 2016;**18**(6):613-625

[4] Shiga T, Suzuki A, Haruta S, Mori F, Ota Y, Yagi M, et al. Clinical characteristics of hospitalized heart failure patients with preserved, mid-range, and reduced ejection fractions in Japan. ESC Heart Failure. 2019;**6**(3):475-486

[5] Tsutsui H, Isobe M, Ito H, Okumura K, Ono M, Kitakaze M, et al. JCS 2017/JHFS 2017 guideline on diagnosis and treatment of acute and chronic heart failure—Digest version. Circulation Journal. 2019;**83**(10):2084-2184

[6] Toback M, Clark N. Strategies to improve self-management in heart failure patients. Contemporary Nurse: A Journal for the Australian Nursing Profession. 2017;**53**(1):105-120

[7] Fowler S. Improving community health nurses' knowledge of heart failure education principles: A descriptive study. Home Healthcare Nurse. 2012;**30**(2):91-101

[8] Suskin N, Sheth T, Negassa A, Yusuf S. Relationship of current and past smoking to mortality and morbidity in patients with left ventricular dysfunction. Journal of the American College of Cardiology. 2001;**37**(6):1677-1682

[9] Wilhelmsen L, Rosengren A, Eriksson H, Lappas G. Heart failure in the general population of men—Morbidity, risk factors and prognosis. Journal of Internal Medicine. 2001; **249**(3):253-261

[10] Li Y, Fang J, Li M, Luo B. Effect of nurse-led hospital-to-home transitional care interventions on mortality and psychosocial outcomes in adults with heart failure: A meta-analysis. European Journal of Cardiovascular Nursing. 2021 (Online ahead of print)

[11] Zhao Q, Chen C, Zhang J, Ye Y, Fan X. Effects of self-management interventions on heart failure: Systematic review and meta-analysis of randomized controlled trials. International Journal of Nursing Studies. 2020;**110**:103689

[12] Jaarsma T, Cameron J, Riegel B, Stromberg A. Factors related to self-care in heart failure patients according to the middle-range theory of self-care of chronic illness: A literature update. Current Heart Failure Reports. 2017;**14**(2):71-77

[13] Sano M, Majima T. Self-management of congestive heart failure among elderly men in Japan. International Journal of Nursing Practice. 2018;**24**(Suppl 1):e12653

[14] Lee KS, Moser DK, Pelter MM, Nesbitt T, Dracup K. Self-care in rural residents with heart failure: What we are missing. European Journal of Cardiovascular Nursing: Journal of

The Working Group on Cardiovascular Nursing of the European Society of Cardiology. 2017;**16**(4):326-333

[15] Sevilla-Cazes J, Ahmad FS, Bowles KH, Jaskowiak A, Gallagher T, Goldberg LR, et al. Heart failure home management challenges and reasons for readmission: A qualitative study to understand the Patient's perspective. Journal of general. Internal Medicine. 2018;**33**(10):1700-1707

[16] Riegel B. A mixed methods study of symptom perception in patients with chronic heart failure. Heart & Lung. 2018;**47**(2):107-114

[17] Lee CS, Mudd JO, Hiatt SO, Gelow JM, Chien C, Riegel B. Trajectories of heart failure self-care management and changes in quality of life. European Journal of Cardiovascular Nursing. 2015;**14**(6):486-494

[18] Goldman L, Hashimoto B, Cook EF, Loscalzo A. Comparative reproducibility and validity of systems for assessing cardiovascular functional class: Advantages of a new specific activity scale. Circulation. 1981;**64**(6):1227-1234

[19] Izawa H, Yoshida T, Ikegame T, Izawa KP, Ito Y, Okamura H, et al. Standard cardiac rehabilitation program for heart failure. Circulation Journal. 2019;**83**(12):2394-2398

Chapter 2

The Dialogue between the Patient's Educational Needs and the Knowledge Transmitted by Nurses: The Case of the Transplanted Renal Patient

Dilar Costa, Joana Matias and Filipa Aguiar

Abstract

Health education has been on the horizon of nursing professionals for decades. The design and development of new education programmes allied to the processes of ageing and chronic diseases have been sought after. In the twenty first century, the need to develop 'performant' policies that lead policymakers, health professionals and civil society to move towards new management of chronic disease marked by citizens' participation in decisions regarding their health and control of the management of their health condition has accelerated the urgency of citizen-centred health care and education programmes tailored to their needs, preferences, values, and condition. In this paper, we explore what has been done around patient education by nursing professionals and the results achieved. We observe a positive scenario where the patient is seen as an active partner, which leads to the integration of a new perspective, assisted and participatory disease management. There is still a need for more structured and systematised education programmes and training for health professionals involved in this process.

Keywords: renal recipients, renal transplantation, education, patient education, nurse, self-efficacy, knowledge

1. Introduction

A closer look at health education programmes shows a panoply of studies focusing on this issue and their influence on citizens' skills and abilities by giving them the tools for learning, taking into consideration their personal needs and problems.

Over time, perspectives and approaches have changed as health systems have evolved. The ageing population and the increase in chronic diseases have put health services under enormous pressure and generated the need to rethink supply in relation to demand. In the context of economic and social modernisation, which has led to an increase in the well-being of one and all, we have seen infectious diseases under control, the infant mortality rate quite low and the death rate diminished. In this vision, resplendent with a better future, life expectancy increased significantly and with it, the proportion of elderly people in the population increased. This accelerated process of economic, social and health changes has considerably improved the living conditions and quality of life of the populations. We are therefore witnessing an increase in chronic diseases, many of which are the cause of high morbidity and mortality [1].

Many of these chronic diseases require long-term care, which contributes to increased healthcare expenditure. Associated with these issues are the high disability rates that affect the living conditions of this group of people.

The dividends of the growth of the elderly population and the conquests in the field of health have allowed the profound transformation of the condition of the population in general and the elderly group in particular. The State maintains support to eliminate social insecurity and ensure the population's conditions of subsistence in economic, social and health care terms [2].

Despite the complexity of this point, people are living longer with chronic diseases and disabilities and health systems are facing budgets under increasing pressure, so societies have sought solutions in order to guarantee the accessibility of their citizens to health care and, at the same time, the survival of health systems. Patient-centred care is thought to be the way forward. As a coordinated care process tailored to people's needs, it supports the development of people's knowledge, skills and confidence to manage their health in an informed way, i.e., the process promotes the means for self-care practice [3].

Now, more and more health systems advocate the path of patient empowerment and involvement, although there are divergences between countries on this issue, and the path of patient dependence on health professionals has not yet been fully abandoned. The issue is also related to rising healthcare costs due to the longevity of the population and the rising prices of drugs and technology, with the system at risk of collapse if the pre-existing models of care are maintained [4].

For Coulter & Magee, the collapse can be avoided if patient autonomy and involvement are encouraged. The emphasis on patient autonomy encourages citizens to adopt healthy lifestyles and consequently puts less pressure on health systems [5].

This idea takes us to the heart of the debate about moving healthcare from doing 'for' people to 'with' people, including them in decisions and making them accountable for their health. As part of this shift towards patient-centred care, health professionals need to focus on educating patients, their conditions and treatment options, and inviting them to participate and be involved in their health care.

The interest in health education results from the articulation of all these elements, longevity of the population that conditions a higher prevalence of chronic diseases, often disabling, related to lifestyles.

Thus, logic of the need to empower people to learn to take care of themselves throughout their lives underlies the process. The Declaration of Alma-Ata itself, resulting from the conference held by the World Health Organisation, underlines that 'People have the right and the duty to participate, individually and collectively, in the planning and execution of health care' ([6], p. 92).

In this declaration, health education is inscribed as the first priority for promoting tools to improve the health conditions of populations and meet their needs.

What happens is that, as seen previously, not all countries show changes in the way they provide care, still maintaining the characteristics of the past, despite the efforts to dialogically involve the patient in decision-making processes [4].

As we know, one of the goals of patient-centred care is to integrate the patient as a partner in healthcare. The success of this partnership depends on professionals taking patients' preferences into account. It is necessary to understand the philosophy of 'patient-centred care'. Can one have patient-centred care while excluding the patient from the process? These are two antinomic terms that cannot coexist simultaneously. The idea is to understand patients' preferences and support them in making decisions that meet those preferences [7].

As patient-centred care is a participatory process, which recognises the role of patients and their ability to assess and determine their needs, the voice of the professionals is not expected to be the privileged element for decisions on treatment/health care.

The reference to education, carried out in health facilities, aims to establish collaboration between the health team and patients in order to increase their effectiveness in relation to their needs and to support them in mobilising knowledge and skills in favour of disease management.

A brief historical review observes different trajectories related to the context of each era, which marked the way in which health systems developed healthcare.

In the 1960s and 1970s, the doctor was the authority, and the patient was a passive person, from whom no active participation in decision-making on health-related issues was expected. The process had as its structuring element a logic of domination/submission in which it was the professional who decided, without taking into account the patient's wishes and preferences, the latter conforming to the former's decisions [8].

Medical power prevailed as the dominant power, medical knowledge as central knowledge and patient knowledge as lay knowledge [9].

In response to the medical-centric model, various movements advocating the rights and interests of patients were set up, thus becoming a driving force for the defence of patients in their most diverse expressions. In the face of such movements, a new development process began from which the contours for a model transition were outlined, medical intervention has been extended to other spheres of social life and health professionals are no longer the only people involved in treating patients [10].

In the 1980s, patient education goes further by focusing on the totality of the patient's interests and the completeness of the patient's values. Several factors converged for this to happen, like the emergence of chronic diseases, the paradigm shift from the biomedical model to the holistic model in health care, the influence of ethics in health care, patients' dissatisfaction with health care, and the call for more information and participation in decisions related to their health [11].

At a political level, macro-trends were registered in the emerging model of people's information and education, the right of access to information, participation, and quality of health care, through systemic and contingent interaction in the face of the change of rethinking health care and the involvement of people who are consumers of health care. In this framework, a new ingredient is added, embodied in the application of technology to education programmes. Thus, education programmes have to be rethought and health organisations have to become organisations that listen to the future, using what can be called holistic teaching-learning systems [12].

In the 1990s, this trend continued, the paternalistic model was abandoned, and the patient became responsible for decisions regarding his/her health. The new logic led to a displacement of the central spaces of professional/patient interaction from the macrosocial, led by the health organisations, to the microsocial space, i.e., to the patient's home, because the patient's life takes place mostly outside the spaces of the health organisations, with daily behavioural self-regulation becoming of indisputable importance in the treatment results. Thus, a model for teaching and training self-regulation behaviours based on a dialogue of equals between health professionals and patients was established [13].

In addition to the patient's involvement, the participation of their wider social network, such as spouse, children, friends, etc., should also be considered. Another relevant factor at this stage is the Internet, which has become a common space and source of information for patients.

The twenty first century, in the field of health, is characterised not only by the increase in chronic diseases but also by multiple comorbidities that complicate treatment and health costs. With this scenario in mind, a global collective project is considered important in health education, which implies the constitution of expressive solidarities between health systems and citizens, in order to act on a large scale and allow the development of integrated education programmes. Going back to Delors when he said that education, and in this particular case health education, is the treasure or the entrance to the twenty first century, it is considered that education is an essential dimension for well-being and for the development of all the person's capabilities [14].

The World Health Organisation's definition of health had already introduced these aspects by extending the concept to the psychological and social dimension of the individual in addition to the biological dimension [15].

It is for this reason that the holistic model is recognised and valued by all. Thus, it is necessary to consider the person and their needs and establish with them the actions that allow them to acquire knowledge and skills to change behaviours, with a view to a healthier lifestyle [16].

The first problem that arises is to determine whether there is currently a change of perspective and attitudes on the part of health systems/health professionals regarding patient education.

It is clear that the main figure in health education is the patient, it seems unequivocal that without autonomy there is no learning. It is important to remember that the person is the protagonist of his/her life project, the active agent of his/her educational process and state of health. Consequently, a relationship is established between illness and lifestyles in addition to other factors such as gender, family structure, environment, and socio-economic conditions [17].

The second question relates to the nature of the health education programmes promoted by nurses to kidney transplant patients. The hypothesis considered is the following: the programmes organised to inform the dialysis patient about waiting list, and to empower them about transplant process, those mobilised around other issues such as daily life management, medication, complications, rejection, and quality of life [18–24].

The object, scope and practices regarding the teaching-learning process change according to the stage the patient is at, i.e., whether the focus is on the pre-transplant or post-transplant period.

Our starting point is post-transplantation. The aim is to analyse in-depth the various education programmes developed in this field of knowledge, identifying their most visible aspects and characteristics. It is, above all, a panoramic survey of the most striking aspects of education programmes in the field of post-transplantation.

Self-determination, motivation, and free choice are important concepts in patient education. The person assumes an active role in this process, through the choices they make, and their accountability for the decisions made. In other words, he/she is free to decide from a range of possible choices. Health professionals involved in this process should bear these aspects in mind because they are extremely important. They should identify the difficulties and constraints that the person faces on a daily basis and promote the means and tools to overcome them [25, 26].

The subjectivity, personal experience, situational, social, economic, cultural, temporal and spatial-geographic factors of the patients are also aspects to be considered by health professionals due to their influence on the teaching-learning process [27].

Health education implies the recognition and identification of the person's symbolic frames, which help professionals to understand their decisions and alert them to the need to anticipate consequences that could be disastrous for them.

In this context, we propose to make an incursion to the studies carried out in this field and dissect the key points of the various education programmes. It seems important to identify the various models and education programmes aimed at transplanted renal patients, not only to verify the differences and similarities but also to disseminate the information already produced towards the transformation of practices.

Underlining the relevance of health education in patient empowerment and self-efficacy, it is essential to define the concept, explore the education programmes implemented in the area of post-renal transplantation and identify their contributions to patient learning.

Before advancing with the proposed objectives, another aim was added: to highlight the nurses' role in this process. Having said this, we now move on to the next section.

2. Health education: defining a concept

The concept of health education has changed over time. In fact, it is an expanding and evolving field. Several authors have defined the concept, and the analysis of some of these definitions allows us to verify the presence of common aspects, such as the cognitive (knowledge), and behavioural dimensions.

The role of the person and the community in advocating for their health is also introduced. Other aspects highlighted were the combination of teaching methods, the introduction of the term 'facilitating', which emphasises the role of the educator as a facilitator of behaviour change, as well as the reference to the participation of the patient in behaviour change towards the adoption of healthy behaviours [26].

What is health education:

> *"All intentional activities leading to learning related to health and disease [...], producing changes in knowledge and understanding in ways of thinking. It can influence or clarify values, provide changes in beliefs and attitudes, facilitate the acquisition of skills, and also lead to changes in behaviour and lifestyles" ([26], p. 25) (1st ed.).*

Whitehead and colleagues health education is:

> *"An activity that seeks to inform the individual about the nature and causes of health/disease and the individual's level of personal risk associated with their lifestyle-related behaviour. Health education seeks to motivate the individual to accept a process of behaviour change through the direct influence of their value, belief and attitude systems, where it is deemed that the individual is particularly at risk of or has already been affected by illness/disease or disability" ([28], p. 313).*

Both definitions bring together essential factors of health education, namely, to inform, motivate, change, and facilitate, aiming at the acquisition of skills and knowledge to change behaviours and lifestyles that are unhealthy for the person.

In this sense, health education is a teaching and learning process focused on wellbeing, prevention and health promotion. The main focus is on changing and improving health behaviours. It is very similar to patient education, but in this case, the focus is on assessment, diagnosis, and the individual needs of the person. In both approaches, patients take a more active and informed role in decisions related to their health. The role of health professionals is to support the patient in this journey.

This clearly refers to the World Health Organisation's definition of health education: "The process which enables populations to exercise much greater control over their health and to improve it" [15].

In this field, three generations of health education have emerged alongside socio-political changes and risk factors: the first generation, based on information and inspired by the biomedical model, the patient should follow the doctor's indications and recommendations; the second generation, centred on behaviour, takes into consideration the need to reduce high morbidity and mortality due to unhealthy lifestyles, while information is only part of the process; the third generation takes participation as the main focus and advocates alternatives for social change, given that not everything depends on the people [29].

Several models support the many perspectives of health education; however, we will only refer to some of these models because they go beyond the scope of this work.

The medical model belongs to the first generation and is characterised by the mechanistic view of medicine, which sees the body as a machine whose parts need to be repaired. It is associated with the authoritarian and paternalistic line of medicine.

The Health Beliefs Model assumes that people act if they perceive (i) they are susceptible to the disease-health condition (ii) the condition would seriously affect their lives (iii) the benefits of their action outweigh the difficulties and (iv) they can perform the action. It means that the person's behaviour is influenced by their beliefs [30].

The Diagnostic Assessment of Predisposing Factors, Reinforcers, Facilitators and Educational Causes Model is used to diagnose and plan educational practices, based on the analysis of the predisposing, facilitating, and reinforcing factors of behaviour, and should be combined with behaviour change models [31].

The Critical and Participatory Models present the proposal of social change and integrate the dialectical interaction between people and their context, promoting the participation of the person and the group [26].

The Empowerment Model seeks to develop the person's capacity to control their health status in their environment. The model seeks to develop life skills, such as decision-making and problem solving, so that the person can take control of their own life. People are encouraged to develop critical thinking and to create critical awareness. Creating critical awareness implies that the person is empowered in their beliefs, feelings, and skills. The model argues that the targets of education are people in general, health professionals and others involved in social and environmental change resulting from political pressures. The main aim is to maximise genuine and voluntary choice. The model also stresses that it does not matter what choice a person makes, as long as it is a rational choice [26].

3. Health education: the dialectic between professionals and patients

Worldwide, citizens' participation in health issues has gained relevance, as has the recognition that it is important to invest in each citizen's ability to make informed decisions about their health throughout their life trajectory.

The current Health System is anchored on a patient-centred model of care, a model that focuses on patients' needs, concerns and subjective experience of illness. The first agent to play an active role is precisely the patient. The new role advocated for those seeking healthcare is that of a person who collaborates with healthcare professionals on decisions related to their health and evaluates the results achieved [27, 32].

Patient education is established in a dialectic between health professionals and the patient/caregiver. Different health professionals are involved in this process, but, in this particular case, the nurse's role stands out as particularly important. Health education and patient education are at the core of nursing practice. Nurses make a difference by helping patients and their families to maintain their health, while sharing knowledge, clarifying daily issues, and training patients/caregivers to cope with illness [33].

The teaching-learning process occurs due to an unmet need. This implies that both, professional and patient, establish a dialogue. The latter indicates to the former, implicitly or explicitly, what their learning needs, preferences and conditions are and, based on this information, both outline teaching and/or training plan that meets the outlined goals [27].

The holistic philosophy of nursing care gives nurses a crucial role in patient education. It is precisely within this framework that the key principles that characterise patient education are highlighted: involvement, knowledge, values, and preferences. This ends up objectively and subjectively delimiting the horizons of the new millennium, whose starting point is the investment in the person, promoting the development of their talents and abilities and the opportunity to practice them. The ultimate goal is to prepare the patient/caregiver for his or her return to family and society [27].

From this perspective, it is important to identify the contributions of education to patient self-efficacy.

The literature shows multiple benefits resulting from patient teaching-learning, such as the reduction of anxiety, the patient's satisfaction with health care, the reduction of the incidence of complications, and the accountability for self-care. It is a process that promotes high degrees of skills and multiple functional versatility, enhancing autonomy, creativity, and empowerment [34–36].

On the other hand, through education and training, it is possible to promote adjustment and adaptability to the new condition. Success results from the promotion of its potential benefits and positive reinforcement. It is evident that the dialectics established between the nurse and the patient/caregiver will tend to positively reinforce the learning and, consequently, promote the development of competencies, knowledge, skills and abilities. However, it is necessary to consider other requirements, such as continuity and follow-up to avoid possible paradoxical effects, especially unlearning and non-adherence to long-term care [37].

For some authors, people are always looking for an opportunity to learn cognitive (knowledge) and instrumental daily living skills that will enable them to cope with new situations, of which illness and hospitalisation fall into this situation.

The absence of health education during the patient's hospitalisation contributes to their dissatisfaction with the health system [37].

Despite the predictable coexistence of the various benefits of patient education promoted by nurses in health organisations, other factors submerge and condition the implementation of the intervention or its effectiveness, such as the shortage of nurses, work overload, organisational culture and low rates of patient compliance [38].

While it is expected in the new system that people will care more for themselves, the efficiency of teaching resources to ensure that learning is adequate and makes patients and carers competent and confident to 'care at home' has not been fully ensured [30].

In fact, the greater or lesser success of any health education process may be related to the way education programmes are designed and administered in different health institutions. Little is known about how this process is carried out by health professionals. This implies the evaluation of possible deviations, in order to try to maintain congruence between the professionals involved in this process [30].

For the author, inhomogeneity may lead to risks for the patient, such as confusion or loss of self-confidence. What seems to be clear in the literature is that this process does not occur in a similar way.

This fact led to the creation of a mnemonic to assist nurses in developing an educational program. This method helped these professionals not to forget any of the steps of the educational process and to develop the process in a systematic and standardised way. This approach proved to be effective and efficient as it increased the nurses' knowledge and behaviours in patient education [39].

The education programme starts at the beginning, but during the process, steps are omitted that can make a difference in the results obtained, which means that the suppression of any step can lead to the established objectives not being achieved. Therefore, training is considered a key element for the professionals' proficiency in this field [30].

In fact, nurses' education is a decisive factor for the success of teaching. It is not only about the positive impact of education on patient experience, but also on clinical outcomes: decreased length of hospital stay, decreased symptoms, increased levels of knowledge and improved levels of patient satisfaction [40, 41].

There is a consensus in the literature that patient education is beneficial to both parties, patients and healthcare, but for education to be effective healthcare professionals need resources and skills to provide it [38, 40].

As a personal development factor, education should be seen as an active component in disease management, which does not seek a simple transmission of knowledge, disconnected from the daily life and the patient's needs, but rather as a means to create synergies that allow professionals to accompany and respond to the patients' demands with existing capacities.

This will be achieved, in part, by adopting the same 'tailored education programme'. As the literature shows great variability in teaching programmes for groups of patients similar in terms of pathology and socio-demographic characteristics, it is difficult to reproduce them in different settings [42, 43].

The evaluation of the effectiveness and efficiency of these programmes is also made more difficult due to the heterogeneity of the programmes and the conditions of their implementation, such as the size of the sample, studies carried out in a single centre - which does not allow the generalisation of results—the variability of measurement instruments - often validated only for that study—among other factors.

Nurses face an important challenge: to create a unifying model in their organisations that support a teaching approach based on systematic, integrated, and collaborative learning. A model that allows for its replication in similar contexts.

One of the advantages of such an approach is that with the introduction of technology it is increasingly easy to share models and trends across organisations to educate the patient.

What is understood from what has been said so far is that health education is understood as an essential part to achieve health outcomes such as the empowerment of the patient/caregiver in disease management.

Nurses have a vital role in the teaching-learning process and the hospital, as an organisation committed to developing the acquisition of skills and knowledge, is a privileged space where, individually or in groups, patients and caregivers learn to effectively manage their health condition and act on the factors that influence it.

An integrated and holistic strategy, based on patients' needs, is crucial for the patient education process. In order to better understand this process and, above all, to capture in the literature the education programmes developed for renal transplant patients due to their relevance to our practice, we have analysed the various studies targeting this population and explored the different types of programmes developed around which we will reflect.

4. Education of the renal transplant patient

Studies show that the education of the transplanted patient is a concern of professionals of the different health disciplines and is considered an important element in the sense that the learning that the patient does inside the health establishments does not remain only inside these places, as it also takes place outside these contexts through the transfer of knowledge to solve day-to-day issues.

These processes of articulation/adequacy between what is taught and what is learned and applied constitute an effective mechanism of success for the different intervening parties. For the patient, it represents knowledge and mastery of new skills to deal with the challenges brought by the disease; for the health institutions it represents a reduction in the number of readmissions, complications, and treatment costs; for society, it means rapid integration of the person in family, work, relational and social life.

The above is part of the problem that health education can play in the empowerment of transplanted renal patients.

The literature recognises that renal transplantation, although the best treatment option for the chronic renal patient, can nevertheless represent a major challenge for this population [42–44].

Kidney transplantation determines a path marked by the need for immunosuppressive medication throughout life, risk of infection and complications due to immunosuppressive medication, risk of organ rejection, obesity, hypertension, diabetes, malignancy, etc. [24, 43].

In this context, the issue of autonomy becomes relevant to the extent that the patient needs to cope with many of these challenges brought about by the transplantation. The answer lies in learning skills that facilitate self-care, such as learning to recognise the signs and symptoms of rejection and the need to adhere to immunosuppressive medication [43].

Chronic disease often affects the patient's ability to perform the activities of daily life, a situation that is associated with kidney transplantation. Patients experience emotional and instrumental difficulties after transplantation, which are often a burden for them and their families [45].

Therefore, patient education is relevant in structuring the patient's day-to-day life and in the transition process. The implementation of a teaching-learning approach to strengthening the patient's ability to cope with the transformations resulting from transplantation highlights the nurses' role in preventing complications and promoting the health of this population group. The purpose of the educational process is to promote the skills and training necessary for the patient's return to normality [43, 46].

Education programmes take on different features according to the places where they take place. For instance, in Turkey, transplant units show dysfunctionalities regarding the way teaching is provided to transplanted renal patients. Patient education does not take place in the postoperative period and sometimes only a single education session is offered to the patient at discharge. Follow-up after discharge and patient's adherence to treatment are not assessed. However, nurses are in an excellent position to recommend and counsel the patients at the different stages of the transplantation process [43].

Been-Dahmen, and colleagues evaluated the effectiveness of a nurse-led support intervention for post-transplant patients. The intervention brought together several key elements, such as a holistic approach, assessment of patients' needs and preferences, shared decision-making principles and empowerment. They held four sessions: the first session focused on self-care assessment (a web-based program was created for this purpose); the second and third sessions focused on problem-solving identified by patients, in the fourth and final session, they discussed the progress made in relation to the results achieved, skills learned and other challenges that arose. They also carried out telephone follow-ups. Results showed in the experimental group, problem-solving skills, higher levels of medication adherence and higher levels of perceived quality of life. The authors concluded that the intervention was feasible and acceptable for patients and professionals. However, the small sample size did not allow predicting the potential effects of the intervention on patients' well-being and self-care behaviours [23].

The relevance of an educational programme tailored to the patient's needs is highlighted in the study by Anderson and colleagues. The programme is based on the patient-centred approach and the principles of Academic detailing. Consisting of three educational sessions on medication, rejection and healthy lifestyles. The sessions were started in the seventh week post-transplant and were conducted by nurses from the Norwegian Transplant Unit. Prior to the implementation of the programme, all nurses involved in the programme were trained to better understand the programme. All interviewees showed unanimity regarding the added value of the programme in increasing knowledge and adaptation to the new situation. For them, the patient-centred approach is highly appreciated as it addresses what is important for each person, taking into account the person's situation before starting the sessions. The existence of a programme designed according to the patients' preferences, values and needs are of great importance, as it means developing actions more focused on their uniqueness as individuals. Guided by the goal of reconciling education with personal needs, lifestyles and family context, this type of programme is particularly appreciated by patients and has positive effects on self-care [44].

Lillehagen, and colleagues present the results of their study. They explore how the new educational programme for transplant recipients is rooted in the daily routine of the ward. The idea was to change the way patients are educated. The new programme differs from the traditional by calling for patient involvement, claiming their individuality and differentiated knowledge according to their preferences, values and needs and includes education sessions. It consisted of five individual teaching sessions delivered by a trained nurse. The topics covered were medication, rejection and healthy lifestyles. The principles of Academic Detailing underpinned the programme. Patient involvement was developed through focus groups between the research group, the healthcare professionals, and a representative from the Norwegian Transplant Patients Association. The authors concluded that the patient-centred approach, tailored education and patient involvement proved insufficient when implementing the programme. In response, patients and nurses extended this approach to the patient's world. The context in which the programme was developed presented limitations to its implementation. With all this, they concluded that the tailored patient education programme involves a more complex understanding of practice than mapping patient needs. The contrast between the virtues of the programme and its failure led the authors to argue that in implementing a programme it is important to critically analyse the effects of adaptations, their impacts, and the underlying reasons [46].

The education of transplant patients is a key nursing intervention that integrates information and training. This set of variables circulates, irrigates and fertilises the patient's knowledge, skills and abilities to deal with transplantation. The entry of the patient into the world of transplantation is a particular aspect of the universe of kidney disease, which requires change, alliances and strategies, completely changing the way patients live, work and relate to each other.

Mollazadeh, and colleagues used teach-back training (TBT) to teach kidney transplant patients to acquire self-care skills. The method was applied to kidney transplant patients attending the clinic of an Iranian hospital. The study evaluated patients with 3–12 months of transplantation. The programme consisted of five sessions. The researchers assessed patients' self-care needs using a checklist, self-monitoring, daily self-care behaviours, early detection of abnormalities, coping strategies after transplantation, and stress management. In the different sessions, patients were asked to repeat in their own words what had been taught to ensure that the information was understood. The training sessions lasted 3 months. The results showed that this teaching method (TBT) proved to be effective, with higher mean scores on self-care behaviours in the experimental group compared to the control group. Before the intervention, no statistically significant differences were found in the self-care scores of both groups. The small sample size and its implementation in a single centre do not allow generalising the results to other settings [47].

Hu, and colleagues, describe the effects of an education programme on the transition from hospital to home in a group of kidney transplant patients. The study took place at a hospital in Chengdu, China. Patients in the control group received routine care, teaching given orally on admission and during hospitalisation, and a written medical and nursing summary related to medication, diet, exercise, etc. at discharge. A telephone follow-up was performed by the nurse 1 week after discharge, and for 1 month, reminding the patient of aspects regarding outpatient follow-up and general health issues [45].

The experimental group was submitted to a care transition programme at admission and during hospitalisation. On admission, a booklet on transplant management issues was distributed and the patient received an individual teaching session based on the TBT method. Several assessments were performed, namely the risk of early admission and the patient's drug profile history as a reference point. Educational material was sent online and answers to doubts were sent via WEB-Chat.

During hospitalisation, the patient received information about the preoperative, surgery and postoperative care. He also received a new book, now dedicated to preoperative, surgery and postoperative issues. A session on post-operative care was administered, informing the patient about possible complications and adverse effects of medication. The teaching programme ended with sessions directed at self-care behaviours at home and medication management at home. Along with the individual sessions the patient received a new booklet on these issues. The online educational material and the WEB-Chat for clarification of questions were maintained. At discharge, an individualised discharge plan was developed involving the doctor, the nurse, the patient, and a family member. The post-discharge period was followed by a follow-up once a week for 1 month. The follow-up was carried out in a structured way, using a follow-up form. Patients could contact doctors and nurses via WEB-Chat whenever necessary. The teachings were performed by a registered nurse. The experimental group was better prepared for discharge than the control group and had a lower readmission rate.

Video education was another of the alternatives that some authors found to educate the patient. Authors used storytellers told by 25 patients who had been transplanted for at least 8 months and had success stories of medication adherence. Through filmed interviews, the selected group informed their peers about aspects considered essential for medication adherence. The interviews were semi-structured and guided by a script composed of questions about medication. The final product was the creation of a video based on the theory of planned behaviour and consisting of 11 storytellers acting as role models in the management of medication in daily life. Messages were left in the video to encourage patients to adhere to medication. However, the effects of this teaching method were not evaluated [48].

When aligning the methods of the previous study with the study of Mansell and colleagues, it can be seen that the use of the video to stimulate medication adherence, plus the adherence contract after kidney transplantation, was another of the teaching methods thought to ensure medication adherence in transplanted kidney patients. The effectiveness of the planned strategies was not evaluated [49].

The literature also contains a wide variety of studies on therapeutic adherence in the post-transplant period. Some have used behavioural techniques [50] others supportive interventions [51] and others medication administration aids. What is noted is the lack of a standardised approach to educating the patient or strategies facilitating medication adherence [52].

Given the nature of this work, we do not expect to find unique solutions that will reveal a singular method to teach the transplanted renal patient. The literature consulted revealed a panoply of studies addressing this topic and all of them seek to stimulate the patient towards self-care behaviours within the framework of empowerment.

On the other hand, the variety of themes is extensive, and many studies have a very particular focus. In our analysis, we sought to focus mainly on the studies with broader themes in order to allow for a broader reflection on this issue.

Patient education is undoubtedly considered crucial in the management of transplantation because it is a challenging condition for the patient. Many aspects are at stake, and all are interrelated. Knowing how and when to do it is crucial for a healthy transition and adaptation to the new condition and for the success of the transplant.

This set of reasons may support the thesis that not only patients need to be trained, but also health professionals, so that the teaching delivered to the patient is more structured and facilitates its continuity among peers [53].

While it is true that the variability of programs, as well as the issues related to the sample size, the diversity of the instruments used to assess the patients' knowledge and behaviours in addition to their reliability and validity, does not allow for the generalisation of results. In fact, Urstad, and colleagues analysed nine controlled clinical trials on the effectiveness of educational interventions in the kidney transplant population. The analysis showed that, as a rule, the interventions were not properly detailed, making replication in other settings difficult. The quality of the studies is also questioned due to the lack of transparency and inadequacies in the details of the documentation of the interventions and their effects on outcomes [54].

Another factor to take into consideration is the measurement of outcomes over time because most follow-ups do not go beyond 1 months and therefore do not guarantee their effectiveness on the timeline. Longitudinal studies are recommended to assess whether changes persist over time.

The heterogeneity of the interventions makes a comparison between interventions difficult and therefore limits the determination of the strength and quality of each intervention.

5. Conclusion

Throughout our analysis, we have highlighted the type of education programmes developed to teach kidney transplant patient and how these programmes are delivered in terms of structure, content, and outcomes.

After kidney transplantation, patients are heading towards a new path that requires them to adapt to the changes in their lives [55]. The continuity of the functioning of the new organ is ensured through the adherence to immunosuppressive medication, early detection of signs and symptoms of complications, organ rejection, infections, adverse effects of medication and other conditions present in their daily lives [48].

The literature shows that about 36–55% of transplant recipients do not comply with what may be the cause of organ dysfunction and risk of rejection [56].

The lack of knowledge, skills, support for self-care activities and demotivation represent contexts that are not conducive to learning and participation, thus raising the need for interventional spaces in the organisational fabric of health [56].

As highlighted by Bertram and colleagues, how can one deal with the disease if one does not know how to do it? [57].

The dialectic between patients/caregivers and health professionals is conditioned by the information/knowledge needs of the patient and the holistic view of professionals towards the former. In this context, the value of participation is visible, firstly in the identification of needs and, secondly, in the development of educational programs focused on the patient and the identified needs [27].

Due to the characteristics already mentioned in this study, nursing professionals represent a privileged group in the field of patient education. By designing and managing education programs, they teach patients in a space of negotiation between different actors (patients and caregivers), identify needs, and interact with everyone in the search for solutions and strategies to restore patients' autonomy and empowerment to properly manage their disease [54].

Education programmes are situated in a collaborative modality between the health system and the patients and their family and social system. It requires a bilateral and interactive collaboration. They are designed according to the organisational model of care and can be based on a more traditional model or a more innovative model, such as the patient-centred model. The combination of sometimes differentiated but negotiable interests is important as a privileged form of relationship between the health system and the patient.

Our analysis has shown that education programmes vary between different countries and even within each country they often vary between institutions and within the same institution. Hence the importance of programmes being structured and trained by the professionals delivering them to avoid negative consequences for learners, such as confusion and loss of confidence [30].

Our final message refers to the fact that educating, teaching and instructing are three fundamental and crucial concepts for patient autonomy and empowerment, especially for chronic patients, such as kidney transplant patients.

Underlying this statement is education with the patient rather than for the patient. This is the most effective way to achieve the transfer of knowledge and skills essential for the patient to properly care for him/herself. It is important to remember that nursing professionals assume only the role of facilitators and mediators in the educational process and that the rest of the process belongs to the patient.

Author details

Dilar Costa*, Joana Matias and Filipa Aguiar
Lisbon University Hospital Centre, Portugal

*Address all correspondence to: dilarcosta@gmail.com

References

[1] Roter DL, Stashefsky-Margalit R, Rould R. Current perspectives on patient education in de US. Patient Education and Counseling. 2001;**44**:79-86. DOI: 10.1016/S0738-3991(01)00108-2

[2] Skelton A. Evolution not revolution? The struggle for the recognition and development of patient education in UK. Patient Education and Counseling. 2001;**44**:23-27. DOI: 10.1016/s0738-3991(01)00098-2

[3] Rademakers J, Delnoij D, Nijman J, de Boer D. Educational inequalities in patient-centred care: Patients' preferences and experiences. BMC Health Services Research. 2012;**12**:2-8. DOI: 10.1186/1472-6963-12-261

[4] Dent M, Pahor M. Patient involvement in Europe—a comparative framework. Journal of Health Organization and Management. 2015;**29**:546-555. DOI: 10.1108/JHOM-05-2015-0078

[5] Coulter A, Magee H. The European Patient of the Future. Philadelphia: Open University Press; 2003. p. 304. ISBN 10: 0335211879/ISBN 13: 9780335211876

[6] Geraldes PC. A saúde coletiva de todos nós. Rio de Janeiro: Revinter; 1992. p. 208. ISBN: 978-8585228514

[7] Fotaki M. Towards developing new partnerships in public services: Users as consumers, citizens and/or co-producers in health and social care in England and Sweden. Public Administration. 2011;**89**:933-955. DOI: 10.111/J.1467-9299.2010.01879.x

[8] Hoving C, Visser A, Mullen PD, Borne BVD. A history of patient education by health professionals in Europe and North America: From authority to shared decision making education. Patient Education and Counseling. 2010;**78**:275-281. DOI: 10.1016/j.pec.2010.01.015

[9] Carapinheiro G. Do bio-poder ao poder médico. Estudos do Século XX. 2005;**5**:383-398

[10] Deccache A, Aujoulat II. A European perspective: Common developments, differences, and challenges in patient education. Patient Education and Counseling. 2001;**44**:7-14. DOI: 10.1016/s0738-3991(01)00096-9

[11] Albada A, Elbers E, Visser A. Patient education in Western European hospitals: A comparison of the Netherlands, Flanders, and England. Patient Education and Counseling. 2007;**66**:4-10. DOI: 10.1016/J.pec.2006.12.006

[12] Chang M, Kelly AE. Patient education: Addressing cultural diversity and health literacy issues. Urologic Nursing. 2007;**27**:411-417

[13] Visser A, Deccache A, Bensing J. Patient education: United differences. Patient Education and Counseling. 2001;**44**:1-5. DOI: 10.1016/S0738-3991(01)00111-2

[14] Delors J, Al-Muffi I, Amagi I, Carneiro R, Chung F, Geremek B, et al. Educação um tesouro a descobrir. Relatório para a UNESCO da Comissão Internacional sobre educação para o século XXI. Brasil: UNESCO/Ed. ASA; 1996

[15] World Health Organization. Declaration of Alma-Ata. In: International Conference on Primary Health Care. Geneva: WHO; 1978

[16] Oliveira C. Perspetivas Holistas na Educação para a Saúde. Revista Galego-Portuguesa de Psicoloxía e Educación. 2002;**8**:39-46

[17] Crawford K, Low IK, Manias E, Williams A. Healthcare professionals can assist with managing post-kidney transplant expectations. Research in Social & Administrative Pharmacy. 2017;**13**:1204-1207. DOI: 10.1016/j.sapharm.2016.11.013

[18] Kayler LK, Dolph B, Ranahan M, Keller M, Cadzow R, Feeley TH. Kidney transplant and listing: Development and preliminary evaluation of multimedia education patients. Annals of Transplantation. 2021;**26**:e929839. DOI: 10.12659/AOT.929839

[19] King C, Dan W, Johnstone S. Are your patients ready? Empowering to create their best possible post-transplant experience. Nephrology News & Issues. 2006;**20**:54-61

[20] Aghakhani N, Maslakpak MH, Jalali S, Parizad N. Self-care education program as a new pathway toward improving quality of life in kidney transplant patients: A single-blind, randomized, controlled trial. Experimental and Clinical Transplantation. 2021;**19**:224-230. DOI: 10.6002/ect.2020.0044

[21] Urstad KH, Wahl AK, Moum T, Engebretsen E, Anderson MH. Renal recipients' knowledge and self-efficacy during first year after implementing an evidence based educational intervention as routine care at the transplantation clinic. BMC Nephrology. 2021;**22**:265. DOI: 10.1186/s12882-021-021-02468-x

[22] Klaassen G, Zelle DM, Navis GJ, Dijkema D, Bemelman FJ, Bakker SJL, et al. Lifestyle intervention to improve quality of life and prevent weight gain after renal transplantation: Design of the active care after transplantation (ACT) randomized controlled trial. BMC Nephrology. 2017;**18**:296. DOI: 10.1186/s12882-017-0709-0

[23] Been-Dahmen JMJ, Grijpma JW, Ista E, Dwarswaard J, Maasdam L, Weimar W, et al. Self-management challenges and support needs among kidney transplant recipients: A qualitative study. Journal of Advanced Nursing. 2018;**74**:2393-2405. DOI: 10.111/jan.13730

[24] Hsiao C-Y, Lin L-W, Su Y-W, Yeh S-H, Lee L-N, Tsai F-M. The effects of an empowerment intervention on renal transplantation recipients: A randomized controlled trial. The Journal of Nursing Research. 2016;**24**:201-210. DOI: 10.1097/jnr.0000000000000115

[25] Leal EA, Miranda GJ, Carmo CR. Self-determination theory: An analysis of student motivation in an accounting degree program. Revista Contabilidade & Finanças. 2013;**24**:162-173. DOI: 10.1590/S1519-70772013000200007

[26] Carvalho A, Carvalho G. Educação para a saúde: Conceitos, práticas e necessidades de formação. Loures: Lusociência; 2006. p. 168. ISBN: 972-8930-22-4

[27] Antunes MCP. Promoção e educação para a saúde: A participação comunitária como proposta metodológica. In: Educação para a saúde no século XXI: Teorias, Modelos e Práticas. Évora: Centro de Investigação em Educação e Psicologia da Universidade de Évora; 2008

[28] Whitehead D. Health promotion and health education: Advancing the concepts. Journal of Advanced Nursing. 2004;**47**:311-320. DOI: 10.111/j.1365-2648.2004.03095.x

[29] Figueroa IV, Farías MV, Alfaro NA. Educacíon para la salud: La importancia del concepto. Revista de Educación y Desarrollo. 2004;**1**:143-148

[30] Redman BK. A Prática da Educação para a Saúde. 9th ed. Lusociência: Loures; 2003

[31] Santos VL. Marco conceptual de educacíon para la salud. In: Osuna AF, editor. Salud Pública y Educacíon para la Salud. Barcelona: Masson; 2000. pp. 341-353

[32] The Health Foundation. Person-Centred Care Made Simple. London: The Health Foundation; 2016

[33] Dumit N. Role of the nurse as educator: Patient teaching. Revue de Rescherche Scientifique de L'Université Antonine. 2017;**6**:61-69

[34] Seyedin H, Goharinezhad S, Vatankhah S, Azmal M. Patiente education process in teaching hospitals of Theran University of Medical Sciences. Medical Journal of the Islamic Republic of Iran. 2015;**8**:8-17

[35] Blankenship CS, Tortella BJ, Bruno M. Be empowered, a speciality pharmacy education program for hemophilia B patients, impaxts adult join bleeds and pediatric use of rice. Journal of Managed Care Pharmacy. 2014;**20**:151-158. DOI: 10.8553/jmcp.2014.20.2.151

[36] Mersal FA, Abd-El Sattar Aly R. Effect of paient education on coping, quality of life, knowledge, and self-efficacy of kidney recipien te patients. American Journal of Nursing Science. 2014;**3**(5):78-86. DOI: 10.11648/j.ajns.20140305.14

[37] Fereidouni Z, Sarvestani RS, Hariri G, Kuhpaye SM, Amirkhani M, Kalyani MN. Moving into action: The master key to patient education. The Journal of Nursing Research. 2019;**27**:1-8. DOI: 10.1097/jnr.0000000000000280

[38] Moonaghi HK, Zeydi AE, Mirhaghi A. Patient education among nurses: Bringing evidence into clinical applicability in Iran. Investigación y Educación en Enfermería. 2016;**34**:137-151. DOI: 10.17533/udea.iee.v34n1a16

[39] Page C, Cordon C, Wong J. Evaluation the effectiveness of a mnemonic to guide staff when providing patient education to autologous hematopoietic stem transplant patients. Canadian Oncology Nursing Journal. 2019;**29**:123-131. DOI: 10.5737/23688076292123131

[40] Xie J, Ming Y, Ding S, Wu X, Liu J, Liu L, et al. Rising need for health education among renal transplant patients and caregiving competence in care providers. Progress in Transplantation. 2017;**27**:180-186. DOI: 10.1177/1526924817699962

[41] Leek RB, Park JM, Koerschner C, Mawby J, Sonnenday CJ, Nunes JAW, et al. Novel education and goal-setting tool to improve knowledge of chronic kidney disease among liver transplant recipients: A pilot study. PLoS One. 2019;**14**:e0219856. DOI: 10.1371/journal.pone.0219856. eCollection 2019

[42] Pehlivan S, Vatansever N, Arslan I, Yildiz A, Ersoy A. Level of daily activities and learning needs in renal transplant patients. Experimental and Clinical Transplantation. 2020;**18**:498-504. DOI: 10.6002/ect.2018.0151

[43] Talas MS, Bayraktar N. Kidney transplantation: Determination of the problems encountered by Turkish patients and their knowledge and practices on healthy living. Journal of Clinical Nursing. 2004;**13**:580-588. DOI: 10.1111/j.1365-2702.2004.00966.x

[44] Andersen MH, Wahl AK, Engebretsen E, Urstad KH. Implementing a tailored education programme: Renal transplant recipients' experiences. Journal of Renal Care. 2019;**45**:111-119. DOI: 10.1111/jorc.12273

[45] Hu R, Gu B, Tan Q, Xiao K, Li X, Cao X, et al. The effects of a transitional care program on discharge readiness, transitional care quality, health services utilization and satisfaction among Chinese kidney transplant recipients: A randomized controlled trial. International Journal of Nursing Studies. 2020;**18**:103700. DOI: 10.1016/j.ijnurstu.2020.103700

[46] Lilhagen I, Andersen MH, Urstad KH, Wahi A, Engebretsen E. How does a new patient education programme for renal recipients become situated and adapted when implemented in the daily teaching practice in a university hospital? An ethnographic observation study. BMJ Open. 2018;**25**:e023005. DOI: 10.1136/bmjopen-2018-023005

[47] Mollazadeh F, Maslakpak MH. The effect of teach-back training on self-management in kidney transplant recipients: A clinical trial. International Journal of Community Based Nursing & Midwifery. 2018;**6**:146-155

[48] Low JK, Crawford K, Manias E, Williams A. A compilation of consumers' stories: The development of a video to enhance medication adherence in newly transplanted kidney recipients. Journal of Advanced Nursing. 2016;**72**:813-824. DOI: 10.1111/jan.12886

[49] Mansell H, Rosaasen N, West-Thielke P, Wichart J, Daley C, Mainra R, et al. Randomised controlled trial of a video intervention and behaviour contract to improve medication adherence after renal transplantation: The VECTOR study protocol. BMJ Open. 2019;**13**:e025495. DOI: 10.1136/bmjopen-2018-025495

[50] Garcia MFFM, Bravin AM, Garcia PD, Contti MM, Nga HS, Takase HM, et al. Behavioral measures to reduce non-adherence in renal transplant recipients: A prospective randomized controlled trial. International Urology and Nephrology. 2015;**47**:1899-1905. DOI: 10.1007/s11255-015-1104-z

[51] Williams A, Crawford K, Manias E, Ellis C, Mullins K, Howe K, et al. Examining the preparation and ongoing support of adults to take their medications as prescribed in kidney transplantation. Journal of Evaluation in Clinical Practice. 2015;**21**:180-186. DOI: 10.1111/jep.12270

[52] Bittner B, Chiesi CS, Kharawala S, Kaur G, Schmidt J. Connected drug delivery devices to complement drug treatments: Potential to facilitate disease management in home setting. Medical Devices (Auckland). 2019;**12**:101-127. DOI: 10.2147/MDER.S198943

[53] Urstad KH, Wahl AK, Engebretsen E, Larsen MH, Vidnes TK, Stenwig AGK, et al. Implementation of a new patient education programme for renal transplant recipients. Journal of Renal Care. 2018;**44**:106-114. DOI: 10.1111/jorc.12236

[54] Urstad KH, Wahl AK, Andersen MH, Oyen O, Hagen KB. Limited evidence for the effectiveness of educational interventions for renal transplant recipients. Results from a systematic review of controlled clinical trials. Patient Education and Counseling. 2013;**90**:147-154. DOI: 10.1016/j.pec.2012.10.020

[55] Mahdizadeh A, Oskouie F, Khanjari S, Parvizy S. The need for

renovation patient education in kidney transplantation: A qualitative study. Journal of Education and Health Promotion. 2020;**9**:154. DOI: 10.4103/jehp.jehp_574_19

[56] Gokoel SRM, Gombert-Handoko KB, Zwart TC, Boog PJM, Moes DJAR, de Fitjer JW. Medication non-adherence after kidney transplantation: A critical appraisal and systematic review. Transplantation Reviews (Orlando, Fla.). 2020;**34**:100511. DOI: 10.1016/J.trre.2019.100511

[57] Bertram A, Pabst S, Zimmermann T, Schiffer M, de Zwaan M. How can you be adherent if you don't know how? Transplant International. 2016;**29**:830-832. DOI: 10.1111/tri.12784

Chapter 3

Role of Nursing in Urogynaecology

Maged Shendy, Delia Marinceu, Mohua Roy, Amar Siddique and Hanadi Dakhilallah

Abstract

Nursing role in urogynaecology has expanded in the modern practice especially with emerging of formulated protocols and guidelines In urogynaecology. Furthermore, conservative approaches and its success in improving patients quality of life is currently led by trained nursing staff, these areas includes pelvic floor training, bladder retraining, fluid intake modification such as explanation of the impact of caffeinated drinks on bladder activity. The adoption of pessary led nurse clinics are well established model in the current urogynaecology with significant improvement in patients flow rate across urogynaecology service provision. On the investigation side of practice, nurse led uroflowmetry and urodynamics are currently expanding with good outcomes for the patients and service capacity. Nursing role in teaching patients how self catheterise is important in those with voiding dysfunction and also prior to incontinence surgery due to associated risk of voiding difficulty.

Keywords: conservative approaches, nurse led pessary clinic, uroflometry, urodynamics, PTNS, Botox injection, service flow, pelvic floor training

1. Introduction

The expanding practice of urogynaecology in outpatient settings has flourished the role of specialised nurses in the field mainly in the areas related to initial assessment and investigations, conducting urodynamics studies as well as initiating the management plans of stress incontinence, over active bladder syndrome as well as running nurse led pessary clinic for managing pelvic organ prolapse.

These are currently established models both in tertiary centres and district hospitals. Further more, trained nursing staff can perform Percutaneous nerve stimulation and diagnostic cystoscopic assessment in tertiary centres.

2. Initial assessment

In the UK, 3.5 millions women suffer from urogynaecological problem however not every patient has symptoms that impact their quality of life and led them to seek medical attention. One in every ten women over the age of 35 suffers a degree of urinary incontinence [1, 2]. Specialised urogyanecology nurse are able to stratify the patient symptoms according to lower urinary tract symptoms groups which mainly are;

Stress urinary incontinence defined as involuntary leakage of urine with effort or exertion, or on sneezing or coughing [3].

Urge urinary incontinence defined as involuntary leakage of urine accompanied by a strong desire to pass urine (void) [3].

Mixed urinary incontinence defined as involuntary leakage of urine associated both with urgency and with exertion, effort, sneezing or coughing. Commonly, one of the two elements are predominant and most bothersome [3].

Daytime frequency is defined when a woman perceives that she voids too often during the day [3].

Nocturia is defined wake at night more than one time at night to void up to the age of 70 years [3].

Nocturnal enuresis defined as incontinence occurring during sleep [3].

Urgency defined as sudden compelling desire to pass urine, which is difficult to defer [3].

Over active bladder syndrome defined as occurrence of combination of urgency, frequency, urge incontinence and potentially nocturne and nocturnal enuresis.

Overflow incontinence defined as involuntary loss of urine without warning or precipitating factor and it occurs when the bladder becomes large and flaccid and has little or no detrusor tone or function [3].

Incontinence due to a fistula which can be vesicovaginal, ureterovaginal or urethro-vaginal fistula [3].

Voiding difficulties includes hesitancy; that is, difficulty in initiating micturition, straining to void and slow or intermittent urinary stream, or post micturition ripples and feeling of incomplete emptying. They are indicative for urethral obstruction muscle, or loss of coordination between detrusor contractions and urethral relaxation [3].

Absent or reduced bladder sensation is usually due to denervation caused by spinal cord injuries or pelvic surgery. It leads to infrequent micturition and a large-capacity bladder, and is often associated with overflow incontinence [3].

Haematuria defined as presence of blood in the urine. This can be microscopic or macroscopic (frank). It is always warrants further investigation [3]

Bladder pain is common with urinary tract infections but also can indicate chronic inflammatory changes that is present in interstitial cystitis where the bladder pain is usually better with emptying [4]

The initial assessment should also gathering the relevant information about; Weight and body mass index (BMI), blood pressure, Signs of systemic disease especially neurological problems and Mobility and mental state [5].

Urinary incontinence and other lower urinary tract has significant impact on women's life starting from a lower emotional wellbeing up to social isolation and planning daily activities around places with toilet availability. There are questioners that assess the impact of lower urinary tract symptoms on quality of life which is a vital aspect in the initial assessment. A well trained nursing staff should be able to analyse such questionnaire [4–9].

3. Basic investigations

1. Urine analysis; Urinary tract infection (UTI) can simulate over active bladder symptoms. Urine strip testing of urine is a cost effective screening for UTI and cases with positive nitrates and leucocytes on strip test should be sent for microscopy and culture [10].

2. Post-void residual check either by ultrasound scan or by catheterisation should be done if there are voting dysfunction symptoms. Post void residuals more than 150 ml is considered abnormal [5].

3. Bladder diary (frequency/volume chart) provides objective method for quantification of fluid intake, functional bladder capacity and voiding pattern. Patient records frequency and times of voids, type of fluid intake and voided volume along with any leakage episodes every 24 hours for 3 days [11].

4. Urodynamic studies

Urodynamic studies include uroflowmetry and cystometry. A well trained urogynaecology nurse specialist can perform urodynamic studies.

Clinically urodynamics are need in the following cases [12, 13].

1. Mixed urinary symptoms (urge incontinence and stress incontinence) prior to surgery for stress incontinence

2. Symptoms suggestive of detrusor overactivity unresponsive to medical treatment

3. Voiding dysfunction with incomplete bladder emptying.

4. Symptoms suggest neuropathic bladder disorder

4.1 Uroflowmetry

The test is conducted by requesting the patient to void on a commode that has urinary flow meter that measures voided volume over time. It is indicated whenever the patient history is indicative for presence of voting dysfunction especially those with recurrent UTI history and patients with over active bladder symptoms and voiding dysfunction symptoms prior starting anticholinergic medications as they can lead to urine retention as side effects. It is also important to consider uroflometry as preliminary test prior cystometry studies test in patients who have voiding dysfunction symptoms and considered for surgery for prolapse or stress incontinence as they would be at high risk postoperatively [14].

Normal finding includes a voided volume of more than 150 ml voided over 16 seconds with maximum flow rate above 15 ml/sec with smooth bell shape curve.

4.2 Cystometry

It is a test involving placement of catheter in the bladder that measures the intravesical pressure (Pves) and catheter in the vagina or the rectum that measures (Pabd). The bladder is then with water at rate of 50–100 ml per min with an aim to reproduce the woman's symptoms and helps to obtain pathophysiological explanation. The pressure generated by the depressor muscle (Pdet) is calculated automatically by subtraction of (Pabd) from (Pves) [14, 15].

The test is conducted through two phases, the filling phase and then the voiding phase. During the filling phase the patient is asked to mention first desire to void (FDV) and also when they feel a strong desire to void when they would normally go to the toilet at that stage (SDV) and finally when they cannot hold urine anymore and that's taken as maximum cystometric capacity (MCC). Normal bladder function involve FDV at 150–200 ml, SVD at 300–600 ml, MCC at 400–700 ml of the volume infused [14, 15].

During the filling phase the patient is asked to cough regularly every 100 ml or 150 ml to identify any stress incontinence. Leakage without rising detrusor pressure is indicative for stress incontinence. The earlier the leakage is detected in the test the more severe the degree of stress incontinence. During the test patient is asked to report any feeling of urgency and that's counter checked with rising in the (Pdet). Normally during filling phase (Pdet) should not exceed 15 cm H_2O. Rising of (Pdet) beyond 15 cm H_2O indicates detrusor over activity [14, 15].

It is important to note patient with severe detrusor overactivity has less bladder compliance and the MCC is usually low. Those patients can also have very low FDV and SDV and the test at that stage should be done at lower infusion rate of the filing fluid [14, 15].

Filling phase monitoring can identify rising in the detrusor pressure with cough in some patients. Those patient presents with leakage in while coughing and the initial impression from the history is stress incontinence while the urodynamic diagnosis would be in fact bladder overactivity [3, 15].

Once the MCC is reached and patients point out that they cannot hold anymore without voiding otherwise she would leak, fluid infusion would be stooped and patient is moved while the catheter in place to void on a commode with built in uroflowmetry to assess any voiding dysfunction and calculate the voided volume, Maximum flow rate [14, 15].

4.3 Ambulatory urodynamics

The test is useful to consider when the conventional urodynamics fails to reproduce the patient symptoms and the results are inconclusive. Micro tip pressure transducer is used to messure the pressures and the bladder is filled naturally (mostly at rate of 1 ml/min compared to the unphysiological filling in the conventional test at rate of 50 ml/min. The patient carry out her normal daily activities, including those that commonly provoke symptoms. The test availability in vary in various units and that's in itself is a limiting factor for its use [12, 13].

5. Diagnostic cystoscopy

Nurse led diagnostic cystoscopy in outpatient setting using either flexible or rigid cystoscopes has been successful in tertiary centres and it has proved to help service provision and improves patient flow. Patient referred for diagnostic cystoscopy are mainly those having recurrent urinary tract infections, haematuria to exclude bladder stones or tumours, bladder pain to exclude interstitial cystitis and patients with suspected urinary tract injury or fistula. The limiting factors nurse led cystoscopy is the resource availability and training curve required.

6. Management of stress urinary incontinence

Approximately one-half of all women with urinary incontinence complain of pure stress incontinence and 30–40% have mixed symptoms of stress and urge incontinence. Urogynaecology nurse role in managing stress incontinence fall into two areas;

6.1 Advice on life style modifications

Smoking cessation is encouraged as chronic cough exacerbates the stress incontinence. If the patient is over weight, the nurse should provide advice on weight reduction as it would lead to reduction in the intrabdominal pressure and in turn the intravesical pressure. Advice to seek medical help and rectify exacerbating conditions such as chronic cough from pulmonary diseases and asthma and similarly any constipation should be rectified.

6.2 Advice and guidance on pelvic floor exercises

Pelvic floor exercises improve contractility and coordination of pelvic floor muscles. An assessment of pelvic floor strength should be done in women with stress incontinence The pelvic floor musculature consists of slow twitch fibres, which are involved in posture, and a smaller element of fast twitch fibres, which are used during exertion such as coughing. Slow twitch fibres are trained with long sustained repetitive pelvic floor exercises whereas fast twitch fibres are trained with fast powerful contractions. If the pelvic floor musculature is weak, then a pelvic floor exercise improves the muscle strength and endurance and in turn less mobility of the bladder neck on straining and coughing and subsequently lesser degree of incontinence. The pelvic floor exercise are conducted as 3 sets every day of 8–12 contractions. Slow velocity contractions sustained for 6–8 seconds each. The response usually notable in 3–4 months. Additional measures such as weighted vaginal cones and pudendal nerve stimulation may be used [3, 16].

It is important to realise the limitation of pelvic floor exercise in patient with stress incontinence as it helps more the patients mild and moderate leakage with approximate improvement of 30–40% in their symptom profile after completion of 3–4 months course. Further management is needed if no improvement is notable beyond this period [16].

7. Management of overactive bladder syndrome

7.1 Life style changes and bladder retraining

Urogynaecology nurse specialist can provide and follow up with the patient the necessary life style changes that helps to improve the bladder overactivity these include, avoidance of bladder irritants such as tea and coffee and use of decaffeinated brands, lesser use of fizzy drinks such as cola. Reduction or preferably cessation of alcohol intake. Smoking cessation is advisable especially in those with mixed stress and over active components. Fluid restriction to 2–3 a day helps to minimise symptoms of detrusor overactivity [14, 15].

Further more, the nurse guides the patient through the bladder retraining which entails education of timed voiding and systematic delay of voids according to a time table. Starting with an aim for resisting the feeling of urgency and hence the voids every 30 mins that's extends gradually to reach a void every 2–3 hours [15].

7.2 Pharmacotherapy

The urogynaecology nurse provides the patient with information that is relevant to various medication used in the treatment of the bladder overactivity. The medications are prescribed by the clinicians and response to the treatment can be followed by the specialised nurse.

The first line of treating the bladder overactivity is the use of anticholinergics. Block the muscarinic receptors that mediate detrusor smooth muscle contraction and in turn relaxing effect on the detrusor muscle. The response to anticholinergics is notable on 6–8 weeks. They vary in the response based on their on selectivity for various muscaric receptos. Oxybutinin is usually the recommended first line in slow release form. It is none selective and hence has higher side effect profile compared to other variants but it is cost effective. Solifenacin, Darifenacin, Tolterodine, Trospium are more selective on the muscarinic receptors in the bladder and hence lesser systemic side effects. The most notable side effects of antimuscarinics are dry eye, dry mouth, constipation and urine retention. The nurse can check with patient if there is any contraindication for the anticholinergics such as acute open angle glaucoma, mythesga gravis or any voiding dysfunction [14–17].

Patients with voiding dysfunction along with bladder overactivity may be benefit of using mirabegrone which relaxes the bladder wall smooth muscles through stimulation of beta adrenergic receptors and blockage of alfa adrenergic receptors. The main contraindication is uncontrolled hypertension and hence it is important for nurse specialist check the patient's blood pressure prior they start on mirabegrone [15, 18].

7.3 The role of oestrogen's

Postmenopausal women who has atrophic vaginitis are usually having some degree of atrophic cystitis. The use of local of oestrogen to treat atrophic vaginitis helps to reduces the over active bladder symptoms to some egress in those patients. Urogynaecology nurse specialist should highlight such benefits of oestrogen cream to the patient and ensure the prescription given by the clinician is followed by the patient [19].

7.4 Use of botulinum toxin a in the of overactive bladder

Patients who has refractory overactive bladder symptoms are over by clinicians Botulinum toxin A by the clinician and at this stage the patient case would have have had urodynamic studies that confirms detrusor overactivity and have her case discussed in the multidisciplinary team meeting that include urogynaecologist, urogynaecoogology nurse Specilaist, phythiotherapist and may include also a urologist [19].

Botulinum toxin A is an extremely potent neurotoxin and its Intravesical injection under local or general anaesthesia via cystoscopy improves the over active bladder symptoms up to 90%. The most commonly applied regimen is use of 100 units of botox in 20 injection points through the bladder sparing the trigone area. The effect of botox injection wears off in 3–12 months depends on the severity of overactive bladder symptoms. Approximately 5–10% of patients receiving botox injection can develop urine retention postoperatively and hence preoperative teaching of the patient how to self catheterise and empty the bladder twice a day is very important [20–22].

The role of urogynaecology nurse at this stage is participating in patient education about about the botox benefits and help the patient to obtain the relevant information leaflets. Also, nurse specialist should be able to teach the patient self catheterisation and ensure it is done promptly especially in old patients with joint movement or rheumatoid arthritis difficulty who has difficulty in reaching out to able to self catheterise. In tertiary units with cavities of training and supervision urogynaecology nurses can perform outpatient cystoscopic botox injection.

7.5 Percutaneous posterior tibial nerve stimulation

Percutaneous posterior tibial nerve stimulation (PTNS) is the least invasive surgical method used in management of refractory symptoms of urgency and urge incontinence. It is mediated by retrograde stimulation of the sacral nerve plexus. The posterior tibial nerve contains mixed sensory motor nerve fibres that originate from the same segment in the spinal cord as the nerves to the bladder and pelvic floor [23, 24].

7.6 Long term catheterisation

Patients with severe over active bladder symptoms that is unresponsive to treatment options especially with old age and presence of multiple medical co-morbidties can be offered long term catheterisation as an option to improve the quality of life. The catherisation in such cases can be urethral with a narrow catheter attached to small leg bag that can be worn under cloth or suprabubic as this does not irritate the urethra or trigone, and the urethra cannot be traumatised by the woman pulling on her catheter. The use of long term catheterisation can be a potential risk of recurrent urinary tract infection and clinician can prescribe long term low dose antibiotic prophylaxis [20, 22].

The role of the urogynaecology nurse in those cases is to ensure regular catheterisation care for example changing the catheter and adjust the size to ensure the right fit without urine leakage from around the catheter and look for any elements of skin care required in the perineal area from potential continuous leakage and irritation.

8. Management of pelvic organ prolapse

Pelvic organ prolapse is the descent of the pelvic organs into the vagina.The about half of multiparous women have some loss of pelvic floor support however 10–20% of them seek medical advice. The prolapse can be anterior (bladder and urethral) prolapse or posterior (rectal) prolapse or mid compartment (uterine or vault) prolapse. The degree of decent is classified through "The Baden-Walker classification" into four grades [25, 26].

- First degree—descent to a point 2 cm above the introitus
- Second degree—descent to point within 2 cm from the Introitus
- Third degree—descent to a point within 2 cm beyond the Introitus
- Fourth degree—descent to point beyond 2 cm outside the interotus

Prolapse patient presents usually with variety of symptoms including vaginal lump and discomfort, dragging sensation, backaches as well as lower urinary tract symptoms such as urgency and frequency and feeling of incomplete emptying and needing to adjust position to help bladder emptying. Bowel symptoms associated with prolapse vary from constipation to obstructive defecation and needs for vaginal digitation to help bowel emptying [27, 28].

Prolapse has it is impact on the quality of life from physical point of view as well as implications on sexual life [25].

Urogynaecology nurse specialist should be able to assess the patient symptoms and and the assess the degree of prolapse which can be counter checked by the clinician if needed. Provide the patient with leaflets and identify any predisposing factors that participate in making the prolapse worth such as high BMI, chronic cough in patients with chronic lung disease and chronic constipation as well as implication of the prolapse on managing day to day activity and patients sexual life.

8.1 Conservative management

Conservative treatment may be appropriate, although prolapse is a mechanical problem that in general, when patients are fit, is treated surgically [25, 28].

8.1.1 Pelvic floor exercise

Pelvic floor exercises helps limit the progression of mild prolapse and relief milder prolapse symptoms. However, pelvic floor exercises on its own does not to restore normal support and are not useful if the prolapse extends to or beyond the vaginal introitus. It is reported to salivate 42–53% of mild and moderate prolapses up to grade two descent but it is unlikely to have any improvement in patients with more than grade two descent [25, 27, 28].

Urogynaecology nurse specialist should be able to guide the patient through pelvic floor exercises along with the physiotherapist and assess the response in 3–4 months.

8.1.2 Pessary management

Vaginal pessaries offer help to women who decline surgery, who are unfit for surgery, or for whom surgery is contraindicated [29].

Long-term pessary use has a high drop rate because of side effects such as vaginal ulceration, discharge and bleeding. It has been reported that only 15–20% of women uses pessaries as long term approach [30, 31].

Fitting the correct pessary size requires a trial and error. A digital examination allows some estimate of vaginal size. In general, it is best to start with smaller pessaries, increasing the size if not staying in place. Change of pessaries usually with in 6 months if no complications such as ulceration and bleeding. If the vagina is atrophic, topical oestrogen cream should be used twice to reduce the risk of ulceration and bleeding. Pessaries can ring pessaries ranging in diameter from 52 to 129 mm and they placed between the back of symphysis pubis and posterior fornix. They usually help with prolapsed when there is uterus as the cervix fits in the middle of the ring. However patients who had hysterectomy they are more likely to benefit off shelf pessaries compared to the ring pessaries as the shape of those provides better support for the vaginal vault where shape and axis could have changed by the hysterectomy [32, 33].

Urogynaecology nurse specialist should be able to fit the pessaries and change them and identify any ulceration and bleeding caused by pessary use. The nurse led pesky clinic in primary and secondary care is a well established model and proved to be cost effective and reduces patient loads on the outpatients clinics with high patient satisfaction rate [34].

9. Conclusion

The role of specialist urguanrcology nurses are expanding and it is a future prospect talking into consideration the world wide pressure on health service.

The limiting factor are the opportunity of training and initial period of supervised practice. Various units have various set up but the core of practice is nearly standard due to national guidelines from the NICE "National Institute of Clinical Excellence" and IUGA "International urogynaecologist association".

Development local protocol, pathways, SOPs "Standards of operations" that the specialists nurses can follow with involvement of the urogynaecology clinicians and the primary services in the community present the corner stone for steady and sustainable nurse led Urogynecology practice.

Author details

Maged Shendy[1*], Delia Marinceu[1], Mohua Roy[1], Amar Siddique[1]
and Hanadi Dakhilallah[2]

1 North Lincolnshire and Goole NHS Trust, Scunthorpe, UK

2 King Fahad Specialist Hospital, Tabuk, KSA

*Address all correspondence to: mego_marmar@yahoo.com

References

[1] Swithinbank LV, Donovan JL, du Heaume JC, Rogers CA, James MC, Yang Q, et al. Urinary symptoms and incontinence in women: Relationships between occurrence, age, and perceived impact. The British Journal of General Practice. 1999;**49**:897-900

[2] Hannestad YS, Rortveit G, Sandvik H, Hunskaar S. A community-based epidemiological survey of female urinary incontinence: The Norwegian EPINCONT study. Epidemiology of incontinence in the county of Nord-Trondelag. Journal of Clinical Epidemiology. 2000;**53**:1150-1157

[3] Abrams P, Cardozo L, Fall M, Griffiths D, Rosier P, Ulmsten U, et al. The standardisation of terminology of lower urinary tract function: Report from the standardisation sub-committee of the international continence so ciety. Neurourology and Urodynamics. 2002;**21**:167-178

[4] Avery K, Donovan J, Peters T, Shaw C, Gotoh M, Abrams P. The ICIQ: A brief and robust measure for evaluating the symptoms and impact of urinary incontinence. Neurourology and Urodynamics. 2004;**23**:322-330

[5] McGrother CW, Shaw C, Perry SI, Dallosso HM, Mensah FK. Epidemiology (Europe). In: Cardozo L, Staskin D, editors. Textbook of Female Urology and Urogynaecology. Oxford: Isis Medical Media; 2001. pp. 21-35

[6] Price N, Jackson S, Avery K, Brookes S, Abrams P. Development and psychometric evaluation of the ICIQ vaginal symptoms questionnaire: The ICIQ-VS. BJOG. 2006;**113**:1-13

[7] Brookes ST, Donovan JL, Wright M, Jackson S, Abrams P. A scored form of the Bristol female lower urinary tract symptoms questionnaire: Data from a randomised controlled trial of surgery for women with stress incontinence. American Journal of Obstetrics and Gynecology. 2004;**191**:73-82

[8] Rogers RG, Coates K, Kammerer-Doak D, Khalsa S, Qualls C. A short form of the pelvic organ Prolapse/urinary incontinence sexual questionnaire (PISQ-12). International Urogynecology Journal and Pelvic Floor Dysfunction. 2003;**14**:164-168

[9] Kelleher CJ, Cardozo LD, Toozs-Hobson PM. Quality of life and urinary incontinence. Current Opinion in Obstetrics & Gynecology. 1995;7:404-408

[10] Groutz A, Blaivas JG, Chaikin DC, Resnick NM, Engleman K, Anzalone D, et al. Noninvasive outcome measures of urinary incontinence and lower urinary tract symptoms: A multicenter study of micturition diary and pad tests. The Journal of Urology. 2000;**164**(3 Pt i):698-701

[11] Digesu GA, Khullar V, Cardozo L, Sethna F, Salvatore S. Preoperative pressure-flow studies: Useful variables to predict the outcome of continence surgery. BJU International. 2004;**94**:1296-1299

[12] Swithinbank LV, James M, Shepherd A, Abrams P. Role of ambulatory urodynamic monitoring in clinical urological practice. Neurourology and Urodynamics. 1999;**18**:215-222

[13] Radley SC, Rosario DJ, Chapple CR, Farkas AG. Conventional and ambulatory urodynamic findings in women with symptoms suggestive of bladder overactivity. The Journal of Urology. 2001;**166**:2253-2258

[14] Dmochowski RR, Rosenberg MT, Zinner NR, Staskin DR, Sand PK. Extended-release trospium chloride improves quality of life in overactive bladder. Value in Health. 2010;**13**:251-257

[15] Mattiasson A, Masala A, Morton R, Bolodeoku J. SOLAR study group. Efficacy of simplified bladder training in patients with overactive bladder receiving a solifenacin flexible-dose regimen: Resuits from a randomized study. BJU International. 2010;**105**:1126-1135

[16] Dumoulin C, Hay-Smith J. Pelvic floor muscle training versus no treatment, or inactive control treatments, for urinary incontinence in women. Cochrane Database of Systematic Reviews. 2010;**l**:CD005654

[17] Burgio KL, Goode PS, Richter HE, MarMand AD, Johnson TM, Redden DT. Combined behavioral and individualized drug therapy versus individualized drug therapy alone for urge urinary incontinence in women. The Journal of Urology. 2010;**184**:598-603

[18] Cardozo L, Khullar V, El-TahtawyA GZ, Malhotra B, Staskin D. Modeling dose-response relationships of the effects offesoterodine in patients with overactive bladder. BMC Urology. 2010;**10**:14

[19] Cody JD, Richardson K, Moehrer B, Hextall A, Glazener CM. Oestrogen therapy for urinary incontinence in post-menopausal women. Cochrane Database of Systematic Reviews. 2009;**4**:CD001405

[20] Kalsi V, Apostolidis A, Gonzales G, Elneil S, Dasgupta P, Fowler CJ. Early effect on the overactive bladder symptoms following botulinum neurotoxin type a injections for detrusor overactivity. European Urology. 2008;**54**:181-187

[21] RovnerE,KennellyM,Schulte-BauklohH, Zhou J, Haag-Molkenteller C, Dasgupta P. Urodynamic results and clinical outcomes with intradetrusor injections of onabotulinumtoxinA in a randomized, placebo-controlled dose-finding study in idiopathic overactive bladder. Neurourology and Urodynamics. 2011;**30**:556-562

[22] Sahai A, Dowson C, Khan MS, Dasgupta P. Improvement in quality of life after botulinum toxin-a injections for idiopathic detrusor overactivity: Results from a randomized double-blind placebocontrolled trial. BJU International. 2009;**103**:1509-1515

[23] National Institute for Health and Clinical Excellence. Percutaneous posterior tibial nerve stimulation for overactive bladder syndrome. In: Interventional Procedure Guidance 362. London: NICE; 2010

[24] MacDiarmid SA, Peters KM, Shobeiri SA, Wooldridge LS, Rovner ES, Leong FC, et al. Long-term durability of percutaneous tibial nerve stimulation for the treatment of overactive bladder. The Journal of Urology. 2010;**183**:234-240

[25] Beck RP. Pelvic relaxation prolapse. In: Kase NG, Weingold AB, editors. Principles and Practice of Clinical Gynecology. New York: JohnWiley; 1983. pp. 677-685

[26] Prolapse CL. In: Whitfield CR, editor. Dewhurst's Textbook ofObstetrics and Gynaecology for Postgraduates. Oxford: Blackwell Science; 1995. pp. 642-652

[27] Hagen S, Stark D, Glazener C, et al. Individualised pelvic floor muscle training in women with pelvic organ prolapse (POPPY): A multicentre randomised controlled trial. Lancet. 2014;**383**:796-806

[28] Panman C, Wiegersma M, Kollen BJ, et al. Two-year effects and

cost-effectiveness of pelvic floor muscle training in mild pelvic organ prolapse: A randomised controlled trial in primary care. BJOG : An International Journal of Obstetrics and Gynaecology. 2017;**124**:511-520

[29] Wu V, Farrell SA, Baskett TF, Flowerdew G. A simplified protocol for pessary management. Obstetrics and Gynecology. 1997;**90**:990-994

[30] Fernando RJ, Thakar R, Sultan AH, Shah SM, Jones PW. Effect of vaginal pessaries on symptoms associated with pelvic organ prolapse. Obstetrics and Gynecology. 2006;**108**:93-99

[31] Deng M, Ding J, Ai F, Zhu L. Successful use of the Gellhorn pessary as a second-line pessary in women with advanced pelvic organ prolapse. Menopause. 2017;**24**(11):1277-1281

[32] Clemons JL, Aguilar VC, Sokol ER, Jackson ND, Myers DL. Patient characteristics that are associated with continued pessary use versus surgery after 1 year. American Journal of Obstetrics and Gynecology. 2004;**191**:159-164

[33] Ding J, Chen C, Song XC, Zhang L, Deng M, Zhu L. Successful use of ring pessary with support for advanced pelvic organ prolapse. International Urogynecology Journal. 2015;**26**(10):1517-1523

[34] Xu H, Wu W, Wang X, Xia Z. A predictive model of choosing pessary type for women with symptomatic pelvic organ prolapse. Menopause. 2021;**28**(11):1279-1286

Chapter 4

Strategic Leadership in Nursing

Adelaide Maria Ansah Ofei, Theresa Barnes and Yennuten Paarima

Abstract

Managing the complex healthcare facility in a lower middle-income country (LMIC) such as Ghana can be challenging and demands management principles that would enable the leader to be conscious of the significant role of the environment. Nurses and midwives constitute majority of the health workforce, play pivotal role in healthcare delivery, consuming most of the resources in managing patient care, and promote the corporate image of the facility. Nurse leaders should exhibit practical leadership skills that would enable effective utilization of the capabilities of staff to achieve organizational goals and prominence in the environment. Long-term viability and competitiveness of the healthcare system demands cost-effective strategies using organizational competencies to take advantage of the opportunities within the environment. Leadership, therefore, becomes essential by initiating a vision that harnesses the potential of staff and stakeholders to this commitment. To withstand time and change, strategic leadership principles such as setting high standards of excellence, demonstrating exceptional performance, and constantly delivering value are imminent. Strategic leadership in nursing ensures provision of leadership strategies that would enhance effective teams and mitigate existing challenges confronting the health system. The paper finds that nursing as a profession is incessantly evolving and, hence, requires strong and dynamic leadership.

Keywords: strategic leadership, strategic management, relationship management, nursing management, transformational leadership, laissez-faire, transactional leadership, healthcare, leadership continuum, nursing administration

1. Introduction

Managing the health needs of the populace in a lower middle-income country (LMIC) such as Ghana is an enigma, due to the many challenges confronting the health system, particularly, the varied professional groups, increased cost of delivering care, increased workload, and the continuous diminishing numbers of staff. Being the largest group of healthcare professionals, nurses and midwives are pivotal to these issues. Thus, nurse leaders are constantly searching for the "best" approach to facilitate both staff and patients' outcomes amid these challenges [1]. Encountering these challenges and other related healthcare issues, nurse leaders should exhibit practical leadership skills that would enable effective utilization of the capabilities of staff to achieve organizational goals and prominence in their environment.

To ensure the long-term viability and competitiveness of the healthcare system, nurse leaders need a set of guiding principles or search for strategies cost-effectively using organizational competencies taking advantage of the opportunities within the environment whilst avoiding environmental threats. Leadership, therefore, becomes very essential in this approach by initiating a vision that harnesses the potential of staff and stakeholders to this commitment. For an organization to withstand time and change, strategic leadership principles such as setting high standards of excellence, demonstrating exceptional performance, and constantly delivering value.

The administration of nursing staff thus becomes crucial to any healthcare system due to their numbers and essential roles [2]. The phrase "nursing administration" is used to denote a broad range of nursing professionals who are well-versed in the principles of effective leadership in the healthcare industry. It is the art and science of planning, organizing, leading, coordinating, controlling, policy-making and motivating human resources towards the achievement of organizational goals. Nursing administration promotes commitment, cohesiveness, coherence, and direction to the provision of nursing services by encouraging efficiency and comprehensiveness in accomplishing the purposes and goals of nursing. Strategic leadership is sensitive to taking advantage of the core competencies of nursing staff to deliver quality incomparable healthcare.

In today's healthcare market, nurse administrators can highly impact the need for lower prices and better treatment that becomes a daily headline through leading and dealing with a wide range of concerns, such as policy, administration, finances, culture, and human resources. Nurse administrators are multi-faceted professionals who establish objectives and strategies for the departments of nursing and maintain organizational structure and culture to achieve the objectives by the maintenance of stable staffing patterns, selecting and assigning nursing personnel and formulating policies that are indispensable aspects of nursing administration. Additionally, they maintain proper nursing records for clinical and administrative purposes as well as constantly evaluate and improving nursing care of patients with the established nursing standard.

2. Principles of nursing administration

Nursing departments uphold the cooperate values and promote the image and services of the healthcare system. Nursing staff are guided by the principles of excellence in service, excellence in practice and excellence in leadership in promoting competitive advantage within the confines of their immediate environment and beyond. Patients, regardless of their circumstances, have intrinsic value and should be treated with dignity and respect, according to the principles of excellence in service. Patients' rights to privacy and confidentiality must always be respected in the pursuit of high-quality comprehensive care that is affordable and based on cutting-edge technology. Thus, every interaction with patients and their families should be marked by empathy and consideration for the wellbeing of those being served.

The nursing profession is viewed as both a science and an art, with the core values of nurturing and care. The practice of nursing evolves around knowledge (science) which is modelled in practice (art). Compassion and care are fundamental to the profession's principal responsibility: in restoring and maintaining patients' health. Patients' health needs are managed holistically by nurses and other healthcare team members utilizing the models of nursing care. For instance, nurses monitor and evaluate nursing practice through auditing to improve patient-centered care and health education. Continuing education, membership in a professional association, and research are all ways in which nurses can ensure that clients' needs are met, and nursing practice remains competitive.

Nurses, according to the principles of excellence in leadership, should foster a progressive work environment that utilizes current technologies while exercising fiscal prudence to enable the greatest possible standard of healthcare. The health system should be a learning organization that engages research to enhance evidence-based practice. The role of the nurse is to promote and facilitate group decision-making. It is critical that nurses become sensitive to the unique requirements of each patient and promote, commend, recognize, and encourage professional and personal development to enhance the quality and differentiation of service. Suggestions and criticisms should be considered as challenges for improvement and innovations thus, giving room for flexibility and creativity. Equity, fairness and engagement should be employed in all performance and personnel policies to promote confidence, competence and commitment.

Nursing administration through effective communication eliminates misconceptions, misinterpretations and create shared vision, direction, and understanding among staff. Subsequently, it is essential to establish effective control. Control is an aspect of nursing administration that comprises of ongoing monitoring and evaluation of the execution of the plan. Supportive supervision via standard-setting, comparing performance with standards and making necessary corrections to ensure achievement of organizational goals. Effective communication enhances control in the nursing environment. Objectives are effectively communicated, roles and responsibilities as well as resources are distributed to accomplish all activities without any misunderstanding and confusion among staff.

3. Nuances of leadership and management

Leadership and management actions can be initiated with "the goal in mind," that is, outcomes that justify the existence of the organization [3]. Nurse managers at all levels of the health system should strive to improve the well-being of the patients. The nurse manager should integrate the department's vision to the hospital's strategic objectives or vision and focus time on activities that converge energy to the results. Leaders must have the ability to motivate and inspire others to work with a passion for common objectives [4]. When it comes to leadership in healthcare, it is the capacity to get people to work together toward a common objective [5, 6]. Good leaders must help others to overcome obstacles and achieve goals, even when the situation is difficult. Hence, nursing leaders should create a workplace climate that fosters good working conditions to enhance patient and staff outcomes. Organizational goals can only be achieved through management's use of people and available resources.

Management sets plans and budgets whereas leadership creates vision and strategy. Managing practices involve planning, organizing, implementing, monitoring and evaluation, whereas leading practices include scanning, focusing, aligning/mobilizing, and inspiring. Both tasks are accomplished in concert. Leaders in the nursing profession utilize a wide range of leadership and management techniques. Strong organizational capacity enhances healthcare services and long-term improvements in people's health care through continuous implementation of the eight practices.

Nurse managers should adhere to the eight leading and management practices to become better leaders and managers. The practices can be employed in a wide variety of scenarios to increase organizational performance and to maintain performance over time. For operational strategies and reporting systems to reflect organizational priorities, nurse managers should follow best management practices and adhere to these guidelines. Being well-versed in the usage of management systems and processes and being able to meet those expectations are two key characteristics of successful nurse managers. Supportive supervision and monitoring and evaluation mechanisms that provide timely, reliable information are significant in the provision of feedback on performance.

To run the department effectively, nurse managers should be vigilant on the provision of nursing services to ensure effectiveness (the right services), efficiency (services are delivered in the right way), and consistently high quality to meet patients' satisfaction. Successful managers must accomplish these three objectives first. During the planning phase, the nurse leader conducts a thorough investigation of the environment to obtain relevant information. Strategies are then developed for goal achievement through delegating responsibilities to team members while ensuring that members are held accountable for timely completion of tasks and within budget. Nurse leaders also ensure that the plan is implemented by putting systems in place and assigning tasks to the right people, as well as monitoring and evaluating progress to achieve the intended outcomes.

While management systems are fundamental for dependable operations, management alone cannot ensure success. Nurse managers who implement new tools and systems frequently achieve similar results, unless they successfully train others to use them, change them regularly to suit client demands, and manage the organizational framework in which they operate using innovative methods. Effective nurse managers adapt to any volatile setting and inspire others to do the same. These adaptive abilities enable individuals to succeed in the face of difficult circumstances and limited resources. Nurse managers are well-informed about opportunities and dangers, and their direction is transparent to nurses and other staff. Commitment ensues when people and resources are focused on a common shared vision, and workgroups delivered on the promises made by nurse managers. To lead effectively, nurse managers must direct their workgroup's attention toward attaining achievements that meet the requirements and preferences of clients while also responding to the interests of key stakeholders. With complete assistance, nurses who work on the front lines of healthcare can learn to identify their barriers to service quality, begin improvements, and give excellent service to their clients. To maintain support, the nurse manager may also need to secure top management commitment. Below are the eight leading and managing practices that nurse managers can practice:

- Scanning: identifying internal and external conditions that influence desired results

- Focusing: directing attention to priority challenges and actions

- Aligning and mobilizing: motivating internal and external stakeholders to support desired results

- Inspiring: creating commitment and a climate of continuous improvement

- Planning: preparing a set of activities, timeline, and accountabilities to meet goals

- Organizing: developing structures, systems, and processes to support the plan of action
- Implementing: carrying out and adapting the plan of action while coordinating related activities
- Monitoring and evaluating: observing, examining, and assessing progress.

4. Leadership and strategy

Nurse managers have 24-h responsibility for managing nurses, nursing units, and patients and serve as a bridge between the operational and management levels of the facility [7]. They are responsible for creating a safe and healthy work environment for the healthcare staff as well as ensuring that members of the multidisciplinary teams continue to grow professionally and offer high-quality treatment, foster a supportive and encouraging work environment [7]. The nurse manager position is significant thus, requires effective and efficient leadership that is conceptual, technical, and humane.

To understand strategic leadership, it is important to separate the two words, leadership, and strategy. Leadership is a process whereby people are influenced by an individual to work toward the attainment of a mutually agreed goal willingly and enthusiastically [8]. On the other hand, management is defined as "the pursuit of organizational goals efficiently and effectively by integrating the work of people through planning, organizing, leading, and controlling the organization's resources" [9]. Strategy is a matter of doing things differently or doing the same things in a new way, making a deliberate decision to do something different from your competitors, and developing a system of operations that is distinct from those of competitors. To cut costs and improve on-time performance, one needs a system that sets apart us from the competition.

The nurse manager in maintaining her unique position in the healthcare facility needs both leadership and strategy to coordinate the affairs of colleagues and stakeholders to uphold the values and integrity of the facility. Leadership is needed for developing and sharing a sound vision whereas strategy is needed to achieve the vision and position the facility within the environment with an incomparable competitive advantage.

5. Strategic leadership defined

Strategic leadership is the ability to anticipate, imagine, maintain flexibility, and empower others to accomplish strategic change as needed. Organizational development, or the process of delivering leadership and inspiration, is what it's all about. The multifunctional work requires managing via others, managing an entire organization rather than a functional subdivision, coping with change, attracting, and managing people (and intellectual) resources, and being able to actively influence others.

The art and science of strategic leadership go hand in hand. Having an open mind, looking at things from a different perspective and being willing to consider the 'what if possibilities,' as well as the bravery to analyze and weigh the various options, are all part of the art of problem-solving. To be a strategic leader, one must have the confidence to make decisions, implement policies, and convince others to share your vision and work together to accomplish it. Thus, focus your thoughts and take action to bring your goal to fruition.

Strategic leadership, therefore, is the interaction of acting, thinking, and doing or influencing the capability of leaders. Strategic leaders are in all levels of the organization as individuals and teams. Nurse leaders are found in all levels of the health system playing formidable roles for the achievement of organizational objectives. Thus, it is essential to develop them to acquire this role orientation to become strategic leaders to achieve organizational prominence.

6. Characteristics of strategic leadership

Strategic leaders' tasks and responsibilities include leading and managing change and making use of the organization's unique resources to ensure the organization's successful evolution. To be effective, a strategic leader must provide direction to the organization in a way that everyone can comprehend and appreciate [10]. Long-term and often major organizational changes are part of the work of strategic leaders, who have a wide range of responsibilities. Strategic leadership is a learning process that uses a combination of thinking, acting, and persuading skills to move an organization in the direction of long-term success. In other words, strategic leaders are excellent managers and leaders who are continually looking for ways to improve.

Strategic leadership is a continuous process and a cycle. 'It is not enough just to 'think,' 'plan,' and 'reflect', people expect to see things happen. This cycle involves (1) assessing where we are. The nurse leader conducts environmental analysis in the facility, or department to know where they are. The environmental analysis involves both internal and external analysis. The internal analysis includes identifying the strengths and capabilities of staff, resources, vision, mission, policies, objectives, activities accomplished previously, etc. The weakness of the organization should also be identified such as staff and resource inefficiencies, etc. the external analysis will help you to identify the opportunities and threats within the environment. The data gathered from this analysis will then be analyzed. (2) Understanding where we are and want to be – Mission, vision. The nurse leader analyses all the data gathered in step (1) to understand the current situation. (3) Learning how to get there —Planning and using strategies that will continue to define us. This involves critical analysis of the data gathered, studying other successful organizations, and using benchmarks to develop plans and strategies. Again, organization of resources as well as alignment and mobilization of staff. (4) Making journey—Implementing tactics. Implementation starts with monitoring and evaluation together with inspiration. The nurse leader monitors all activities being implemented to ensure the right things are done or take corrective actions where necessary. Nurses are inspired throughout the process to maintain the momentum of implementation thus, encouraging creativity and innovation to enhance core competencies. (5) Checking progress—Current performance. The nurse leader continuously checks all the activities been accomplished to sustain enthusiasm by motivation through acknowledgement and praise. Thus, the strategic organization is all about continually becoming. Strategic leadership involves discovery more than determination and is not reserved for those at the top only.

Essential for nurse managers are the provision of direction, application of strategic thinking for policymaking, a clear plan of action, balance long and short-term goals; develop ownership; build partnerships; leading by example and a succession plan for the future of the organization. This creates a balance between short-term and long-term goals, strategic leadership in oneself and others, making words into action (making the journey), monitoring the progress, and changing course if necessary are all significant for nurse managers. They need to be able to think, act, and have an impact. A nurse manager's strategic strategy is nothing more than that. The judgments and choices that an organization makes when they implement or fail to implement the plan constitute a real strategy.

Everyone, not only the CEO or nurse leader, has a role to play in strategic leadership. A collection of processes cannot adequately describe this never-ending cycle of personal, group, and organizational growth. It aims at helping senior executives and future leaders build and maintain a focus on the 'essential few' factors that have been determined to be most critical to the long-term success and competitiveness of the organization. All these aspects are necessary for organizations to be long-term winners in the face of change and uncertainty and to continually give value to all of their main stakeholders—including society—no matter how challenging the environment. The 'roadmap' is the executive blueprint for moving the organization to the next level of performance and competitiveness. These important performance components should be included.

To be effective, a strategic leader must have transformative powers, act morally and politically when appropriate, prioritize the relationship between the organization and its environment, and possess strong managerial skills. Successful strategic leaders, according to Cousins [11], have specific cognitive and conceptual abilities. According to him, they are analytical, creative thinkers who can thrive in a dynamic and complicated environment because of their analytical, creative, innovative, reflective, and proactive thinking abilities [11]. As a healthcare organization, nursing necessitates leaders who possess these traits to achieve and maintain a competitive edge.

7. Components of strategic leadership

When it comes to effective strategic leadership, there are five key components: (1) Creating an inspiring mission statement and sharing it with colleagues, (2) Developing high-level cognitive activity because developing strategies is hard mental work, (3) Gathering multiple inputs, that is strategy formulation which is democratic, (4) Anticipating and creating a future that involves the invention of a new world, and (5) Revolutionary thinking and action to get things accomplished.

The critical performance components of strategic leadership include the (1) Organization's Business Model which must be designed and driven by the leadership team, who must focus relentlessly on 'doing the right things for the business – not just 'doing things right'. (2) Organizational culture, particularly, the values or beliefs can either be the greatest enabler or inhibitor of organizational performance. (3) An organization's core shared purpose which becomes the 'anchor' that keeps the organization from 'drifting' into danger in the sea of turbulence. (4) Renewal that is the seamless integration of adaptability, innovation, and continuous learning, which is the secret ingredient that sustains the organization's 'vitality', its 'relevance' through time so its 'business model' never becomes outmoded. (5) Organization's vision, which is the destination the organization wants to reach. The organization is on a journey, and it is the responsibility of the leader to ensure that it ends up at the desired destination. (6) Principles of engagement which cover how the organization presents itself to society including such topics as corporate governance, corporate social responsibility, sustainability or environmental programs, ethical practices and more. Over time these principles define and either strengthen or weaken the organization's image and even the strength of the brand. They cannot be minimized or trivialized. (7) Investing in the growth of the organization's human resources. When an organization aligns itself around a goal or vision, it can harness all of the organization's resources to achieve that goal. For the achievement of the vision, it is necessary to include the following elements: critical success factors, performance drivers, key business objectives (KBOs), and the strategies that assist in achieving these KBOs, all of which must be implemented perfectly to achieve the desired outcomes.

(8) Creation and delivery of value to all key stakeholders including society. Values are defined as any of the tangible or intangible benefits that the customer or stakeholder perceives he or she receives from you and would not realize from any other provider. As such it represents an immediate source of differentiation and is also the foundation for building and maintaining exceptional stakeholder relationships. (9) Agility and resiliency; agility involves identifying, assessing, and acting on opportunities (or threats) faster and better than competition. Resiliency involves recovering from problem situations better and faster than a competitor – minimizing the potential 'cost of lost opportunity'. (10) Relationship mastery; this is the capability to build and maintain exceptional and secure relationships with all key stakeholder groups including customers. In times of market turbulence nothing contributes more to the organization's stability than well-defined and secure relationships with key stakeholders. (11) Competitiveness and growth; the ultimate outcome which is driven by the above. There must be also a sensing system or strategic information architecture to support all the above components including a hyper-decision-making capability.

8. Strategic leadership process

The healthcare industry has expanded its understanding of the significance and impact of strong leadership [12]. The healthcare system's complexity necessitates the skills of a capable leader who can bring together medical and clinical practice while also recognizing the needs of patients and establishing a wide range of health services [13]. The primary goal of the healthcare sector is to provide preventive, rehabilitative, and palliative care to a community [14]. The strategic leadership process has four stages: competence, vision, communication, and service.

Step 1—The capacity to meet a specific demand, an honest appraisal of one's skills, shortcomings, goals, and motivating factors, the development of a competency that others respect, and the competency must be recognized by the organization, are all components of competence. Developing exceptional competence requires 10–18 years, and early development of core competence should be prioritized through investment.

Step 2—To guide the organization in the right direction and create a vision that serves as a guidepost. This creates a motivational focus, giving employees a specific goal to work toward. The following are characteristics of a vision: To be imaginable is to have a vision of the future. Long-term interest appeals to stakeholders are desirable. Clear: able to serve as a compass for making decisions. Adaptable: allowing for a wide range of reactions and allowing for individual initiative. The term "communicable" refers to the ability to communicate effectively within five minutes.

Step 3—Included in the list of questions to inquire about the effectiveness of communication is: The vision statement will be communicated to whom? What are all the possible means of communication? We must consider how we can best convey the organization's long-term strategy to our stakeholders. What are the best means of contacting you in the future? What measures can be used to assess whether or not the vision statement is known and understood by the target audience? A vision statement without proper communication is like hosting a party without sending out invitations.

Step 4—Empathy, healing, listening, awareness, foresight, persuasion, stewardship, dedication to the growth of people, developing community, and conceptualizing are among the 10 characteristics of servant leaders highlighted by Spears [15]. The leader-follower relationship should be built on open and reciprocal exchanges of information. Being able to listen and be open to what others have to say is a learned skill. Through good listening, servant leaders recognize and validate the thoughts of their subordinates. Servant leaders that are empathic show that they truly understand the thoughts and feelings of their subordinates. It's all about the help a servant leader gives their followers to overcome their own personal struggles. Servants who are aware of their social, physical, and political surroundings are better able to respond to the needs of their organizations. Persuasion is the ability to communicate in a way that persuades others to change their minds. Focus on the person's capacity to be a visionary for the organization by providing a rich sense of objectives and direction. Servant leadership requires foresight and accountability, while stewardship requires accountability for one's leadership role. For those who want to learn more about servant leadership, these ten traits are an excellent starting point.

9. Relationship management

To complete all four elements of the Strategic Leadership Process, managing relationships is essential. As a strategic leader, you need to manage your connections with your colleagues, executives, and employees effectively. Listening and effective talking are two abilities that can help manage relationships.

Being a nurse administrator or leader necessitates a high level of listening skills. (1) Ignoring is a form of listening in which the listener does not pay attention to what the speaker is saying. (2) "Pretend listening" refers to the practice of paying scant attention to a speaker while doing other things. (3) Selective listening usually occurs in a group setting where one tunes in and out depending on the interest of the verbal cues. (4) Attentive listening is focusing on the speaker and not allowing external noise or potential distractions to interfere with the messages being conveyed. (5) Empathic listening is the most successful kind of listening because it allows you to put yourself in the other person's shoes and fully comprehend what they are trying to say. Strategic leadership in the healthcare industry necessitates that the nurse leader is well-versed in all these types of listening styles to effectively engage colleagues and build trust.

Keys to the effective conversation are (1) Candor: setting up an agenda with one's feelings, beliefs, or ideas. That is the act of being open and honest or frank. Conversations with colleagues should be straightforward and sensitive to their sentiments. (2) Clarity: verbal and non-verbal exchange of wants and needs should be the same and specific. (3) Commitment: agreement on next steps. Nurse leaders should learn to agree with colleagues on the next steps to adopt and be committed to them.

10. Effective strategic leadership

Nursing as a profession is incessantly evolving hence requires strong and dynamic leadership. The complex and dynamic nature of the nursing environment requires nurse executives to leverage the basic tenants of strategic leadership to promote nursing performance and service delivery [14]. It's all about developing a feeling of purpose and direction, which are crucial enablers for interacting with key internal and external aspects in the organization's environment [16]. Strategic leadership, according to Nwachukwu and Vu [17], is based on the ability of a leader to think strategically and see the future to improve the efficiency of the business. Strategic leadership is not only about having unique qualities that allow for the acquisition and learning of new knowledge and ideas but also having an adaptive capacity to effectively respond to the dynamism and complexity of the external environment. Hence, strategic leaders may respond to a changing environment by constantly and tactically adjusting their organization. The presence of strategic leadership is not enough to promote organizational effectiveness as other antecedents can be at play [16]. Effective strategic leadership is a crucial aspect of organizational effectiveness and has been associated with numerous organizational outcomes [18]. Effective strategic leadership can identify the moderation and mediating factors such as the internal and external environmental dynamics, taking advantage of the opportunities and overcoming the threats [19]. Organizational strategic flexibility and sustainability are facilitated by the strategic leadership. This means that a nursing organization's long-term strategic planning hinges on its leadership, in which leaders adopt a common vision of what the organization will become [12].

To be an effective strategic leader, an organization should first determine its long-term goals, strike a balance between internal and external controls, efficiently manage its resources, maintain an effective organizational culture, and focus on ethical standards.

1. Choosing a course of action. Involves defining a long-term goal and a strategy for achieving goals. For the next 3–5 years, strategic direction is articulated in terms of the opportunities and dangers that exist. All organizations need to have a strong foundation of beliefs and a clear vision of what the future holds.

2. Organizational controls that are well-balanced. Strategic and financial controls must be developed and used effectively by strategic leaders. Controls define the parameters by which strategies are to be implemented and the actions that must be performed to change those strategies once they have been implemented. Financial and strategic controls must be balanced to succeed. For strategic executives, the Balance scorecard framework is a way to check that they have created both financial and strategic controls to measure organizational performance Premise is that when financial controls are prioritized above strategic controls, organizations put their future performance at risk. Organizations can use diverse views to attain higher levels of performance when strategic and financial controls are properly balanced. Financial perspective criteria involve cash flow, return on equity and return on assets. Customer perspectives criteria consist of the assessment of the ability to anticipate customers' needs, the effectiveness of customer service practices, the percentage of repeat business, and the quality of communication with customers. Internal business processes perspective criteria include improvements in innovation ability, improvements in employee morale and

changes in turnover rates. Learning and growth perspective criteria also include improvements in innovation ability, the number of new products compared to computers and increases in employees' skills.

3. Effectively managing the organization's resource portfolio. This includes financial, organizational (competencies and capabilities) and human capital. Organizations' resources must be managed in a way that is consistent and supportive of the strategy. They also must be allocated as efficiently and effectively as possible so that each area of the firm has what it needs for strategy implementation. The changing strategy will likely call for the reallocation of resources and the movement of people and other resources from one area to another. Financial resources are managed through the budgeting and resource allocation process. Core competencies and competitive capabilities should be developed in a strategy supportive fashion. Organizations should build their strategy around things they are good at doing and/or become good at doing things that are supportive of strategy. A firm's human capital, which refers to knowledge and skills of a firm's entire workforce, should also fit its strategy. This can be accomplished by hiring people that fit the organization and its strategy, and an effective training and development program. Investments should be made to acquire and develop the firm's human capital.

4. Sustaining an effective organizational culture. This complex mix of basic beliefs, ideas and symbols that are shared throughout the organization, particularly among the employees, have a significant impact on the way business is done. It sets the stage for the organization's strategy-making and implementation. Employees' behavior is also regulated by this method. Organizational culture is made up of a wide range of factors, including its origins. Once established, an organization's culture tends to survive because it hires people who share its values, socializes its employees, and systematically indoctrinates them with the culture's norms and practices. The retelling of organizational folklore and ceremonies honoring personnel who exhibit cultural values. Cultural standards should be rewarded. The robustness of a company's culture can vary depending on how deeply it is ingrained in everyday operations and customs. A company's culture should reflect its strategy to help it become more strategically competitive and generate above-average returns. As difficult as it may be to change a company's culture, with the right strategic leadership, it may be done.

5. Emphasizing ethical practices. Controlling employees' judgment and behavior can be achieved through the application of ethical practices. When it comes to making decisions, they should be a key element of the culture of the firm. It is critical for strategic leaders to set and convey ethics-related goals; continually revise and disseminate the organization's code of conduct; create an acceptable work environment; and utilize reward systems to recognize and promote ethical behavior. Ethical practices can be used to ensure that people are acting in a morally correct manner.

6. Developing policies and procedures. People's behavior is governed by policies and procedures, which are sets of written and unwritten norms and styles of conduct. The standardization of work practices and the specification of the optimal methods for completing tasks can boost productivity. Provide direction from the top-down on how specific tasks should be completed. As a result of their

efforts, important strategic actions are carried out consistently. The kinds and numbers of policies and procedures employed by various kinds of organizations vary widely. There must be a good synergy between an organization's policies and procedures and its overall strategy.

7. Developing reward systems. Effective plan execution can only be achieved through employee commitment if they get incentives. Behavioral control can be achieved in part through the use of rewards. Those who achieve their goals should be rewarded abundantly, and those who don't achieve their goals should not be rewarded. Strategy-based incentives and monetary compensation should be used to motivate employees to improve efficiency and find ways to save money. Distinguishers should recognize and reward those who are creative. Consequently, organizations must reward and encourage their employees in ways that complement the strategy and implementation of the business plan.

11. Strategic leadership and strategic management process

The strategic management process can only succeed if it is led by an effective strategic leader. Vision and mission are shaped by the strategic leadership of the organization, and the development and implementation of strategies are facilitated by the leadership of the organization.

Leadership plays a key role in terms of enforcing organizational strategies. Strategic leaders in an organization work with the strategic vision by formulating strategies, implementing, and evaluating those strategies to achieve the strategic goal [20]. This process is described as the strategic management process. Strategic management is a rapidly developing field of study that has emerged in response to increasing environmental diversities [21]. Strategic management seeks to manage all resources to create and sustain a competitive advantage for a successful future. The focus is to view the organization as a whole and examine the firm's performance attempting to explain why others perform better under similar chaotic conditions. Strategic management emphasizes on decision making, which is a characteristic feature. These strategic decisions are long term and focus on the future of the organization. The distinguishing characteristics of strategic management are its emphasis on strategic decision-making with three key attributes: rare, consequential, and directive [22].

12. Strategic leadership models

All the leadership styles are significant in strategic leadership, particularly when to use each of the styles to realize its usefulness. However, transformational, laissez-faire and transactional leadership are the models used in bringing about strategic leadership. Knowing which styles to use as a nurse leader is important when dealing with a complex work environment such as the hospital where varied accomplished health professionals converge to manage the patient.

12.1 Transformational leadership

Transformational leadership devotes attention to charismatic and emotional elements of leadership which emphasize intrinsic inspiration and follower growth.

This aligns with the needs of today's workforce, who needs inspiration and empowerment to succeed. Working with teams to identify what changes are needed, building a shared vision to guide the change, and then implementing those changes together with dedicated members of the group are all steps in leadership. By changing roles and responsibilities, leaders motivate their teams to put the interests of the organization ahead of their own. It is a process that affects and transforms individuals under transformational leadership. Leaders can also have a unique and reflecting effect on their subordinates and subordinates. The values, norms, ethics, feelings, and long-term objectives of transformational leadership are at the heart of this approach. It also requires assessing the motivations of followers, meeting their needs, and treating them as individuals... Transactional leaders are responsible for the day-to-day operations of the company, whereas transformational leaders are responsible for bringing in new ideas and implementing them.

According to Bass [23], transformational leadership is defined by the impact it has on the people it serves. Transformational leaders, according to Bass, inspire their people to trust, respect and admire them. Transformational leadership is judged mostly on the impact the leader has on his or her subordinates. Transformational leaders inspire loyalty, adoration, and respect in their followers because of the leader's willingness to go above and beyond the call of duty. Due to the transformational leader's ability to foster a sense of personal value in his or her followers, these results can be achieved. They provide adherents with a compelling mission and vision, as well as a sense of self-worth. It is via academic stimulation, idealized influence (charisma), and personal consideration that followers are transformed and motivated to action. Additionally, the leader encourages his or her subordinates to cultivate inventive and unique approaches to question the status quo and modify the environment to achieve success. Because leadership is a continuum from transformational to transactional to laissez-faire, Bass argued that leaders can simultaneously demonstrate both transformative and non-transformative leadership attributes.

12.2 Laissez-faire

Laissez-faire leadership style is when a leader does not provide leadership that allows followers to look after themselves. Subordinates end up with freedom in deciding which policies and methods to adopt. The leader develops the structure of the work and provides adequate resources for work and helps upon requests by coaching or answering questions or supplying information. However, the leader does not participate in workshop discussions or group tasks. The leader again does not provide comments on followers' performance unless specifically requested. As a result of this, employees may become dissatisfied and fail to meet the goals they had set for themselves.

Negative repercussions are commonly linked to leadership, particularly in terms of follower satisfaction or leader effectiveness [24]. Female leaders are more likely to be transformational leaders, whereas male leaders are more likely to be laissez-faire leaders [25]. Those that have a proven track record of excellence or matured employees are most suited for this type of leadership. Using this strategy, more experienced employees become self-sufficient, productive, and impactful. As a result, the approach encourages team members to be creative and original, which in turn aids in the advancement of their careers. Members see a laissez-faire attitude as a vote of confidence in their talents, which gives them more room to grow into self-assured, devoted, competent, and successful individuals.

12.3 Transactional theory

The transactional leader directs attention to the use of conditional responses such as rewards and punishments to acquire compliance from followers. Transactional leaders attain goals by seeking to uphold the status quo, not aiming for advancement, whereas transformational leaders endeavor to transform the future by inspiring the followers. Transactional leadership styles result in increased job satisfaction as well as leader job performance. The leader gets the job done with no commitment from the followers. Because of its emphasis on short-term goals, transactional leadership is more like a management style than a true leadership one. Despite these drawbacks, it can be a useful tool in other settings, such as in the workplace.

As depicted in **Figure 1**, leadership is viewed as a continuum, ranging from transformational leadership, through transactional leadership to laissez-faire leadership. This implies while leaders may have a specific style this may not be fixed, as there are points/situations when leaders' styles may depict traits of the other two. Transformational leaders bring a lot of energy and enthusiasm to the workplace, change and new ideas to management, thus more is achieved. Transactional leaders maintain the status quo and ensure goals are achieved through the routine accomplishment of roles and responsibilities with normal energy, whereas laissez-faire leaders normally lack energy and ideas and bring lethargy to the workplace killing at time enthusiasms. Nurse leaders, in being strategic ought to acknowledge this continuum, understand the peculiarities of a particular situation and know and practicalize the best-fitting approach.

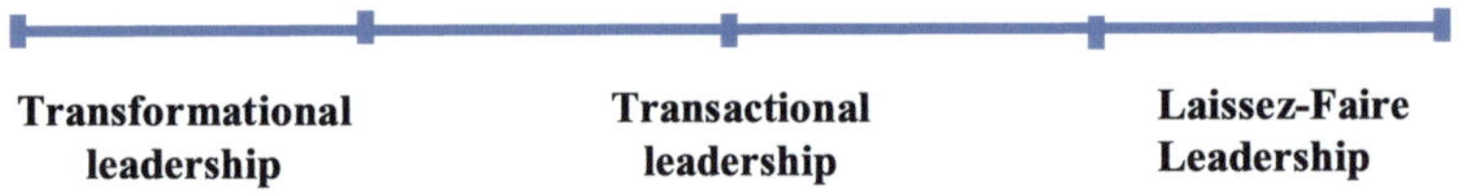

Figure 1.
Leadership continuum.

13. Conclusion

The complex and dynamic nature of the nursing environment requires nurse executives to leverage the basic tenants of strategic leadership to promote nursing performance and service delivery. Leadership plays a key role in terms of making and enforcing organizational strategies. Leadership capabilities and strategies are essential for optimizing team-based nursing and patient outcomes. A visionary leadership approach motivates teamwork and seeks to reach the highest levels of performance possible within the boundaries of nursing practice.

Many studies support the transformational method since it encourages employees to work creatively, exhibit dedication, and meet expectations. Some research suggests combining the three styles in management because each situation necessitates a distinct style. Transformational and laissez-faire methods encourage employees' independence and creativity. When a leader wants to develop new practices and implement them quickly, transactional approach works best.

Strategic Leadership in Nursing
DOI: http://dx.doi.org/10.5772/intechopen.104512

Author details

Adelaide Maria Ansah Ofei*, Theresa Barnes and Yennuten Paarima
Department of Research, Education, and Administration, School of Nursing and Midwifery, University of Ghana, Ghana

*Address all correspondence to: adelaideofei@gmail.com

References

[1] Asamani JA, Naab F, Ansah Ofei AM. Leadership styles in nursing management: Implications for staff outcomes. Journal of Health Sciences. 2016;**6**(1):1-14

[2] Ansah Ofei AM, Paarima Y, Barnes T, Kwashie AA. Staffing the unit with nurses: the role of nurse managers. Journal of Health organizations and Management. 2021 https://www.emerald.com/insight/1477-7266.htm

[3] Covey S. The 7 habits of highly effective people : Powerful lessons in personal change. New York: Free Press, Simon & Schuster, Inc; 2004

[4] Mitchell LA. Integrity and Virtue: The forming of good character. The Linacre Quaterly. 2015;**18**(2). DOI: 10.1179/2050854915Y.000000001

[5] Aberese-Ako M, Agyepong IA, van Dijk H. Leadership in two Ghanaian hospitals in a challenging environment. Health Policy and Planning. 2018;**33**(2): 16-26. DOI: 10.1093/heapol/czy038

[6] Perfecto G, Aquino J. The effectiveness of leadership styles of managers and supervisors to employees' job satisfaction in cooperative organizations in the Philippines. The Macrotheme Review. 2015;**4**(5):18-28

[7] American Organization of Nurse Executive. AONE Nurse Executive Competencies. Chicago, IL; 2015 www.aone.org/resources/nurse-leader-competencies.shtml

[8] Cummings GG, Tate K, Lee S, Wong CA, Paananen T, Micaroni SPM, et al. Leadership styles and outcome patterns for the nursing workforce and environment: A systematic review. International Journal of Nursing Studies. 2018;**85**:19-60. DOI: 10.1016/j.ijnurstu.2018.04.016

[9] Kiniki A, Williams B. Management: A Practical Introduction. 9th ed. McGraw Hill; 2018

[10] Yardan ED, Aydin GZ. Strategic leadership in healthcare. Health Sciences Research in the Globalizing World. 2018:874

[11] Cousins B. Design thinking: Organizational learning in VUCA environments. Academy of Strategic Management Journal. 2018;**17**(2):1-18

[12] Ginter PM, Duncan WJ, Swayne LE. The Strategic Management of Health Care Organizations. 8th ed. Hobeken, NJ: John Wiley & Sons; 2018

[13] Barr J, Dowding L. Leadership in Health Care. 4th ed. London: Sage Publications Limited; 2019

[14] Min S, Jeong YJ, Kim HS, Ha SY, Ha YJ, Kim EA. The moderating effect of self-leadership in the relationship between self-image and work performance of nurses. Journal of Korean Academy of Nursing Administration. 2009;**15**(3):355-364

[15] Spears LC, editor. Character and sevant leadership: Ten characteristics of effective, caring leaders. The Journal of Virtues & Leadership. 2010;**1**(1):25-30

[16] Jaleha AA, Machuki VN. Strategic leadership and organizational performance: A critical review of literature. European Scientific Journal. 2018;**14**(35):124-149

[17] Nwachukwu C, Vu HM. Strategic flexibility, strategic leadership

and business sustainability nexus. International Journal of Business Environment. 2020;**11**(2):125-143

[18] Phipps KA, Burbach ME. Strategic leadership in the nonprofit sector: Opportunities for research. Journal of Behavioural and Applied Management. 2010;**11**(2):137

[19] Ferreira J, Coelho A, Mourinho L. Dynamic capabilities, creativity and innovation capability and their impact on competitive advantage and firm performance: The moderating role of entrepreneurial orientation. Technovation. 2020;**92**:102061

[20] Wheelen TL, Hunger JD, Hoffman AN, Bamford CE. Strategic Management and Business Policy. Globalization, Innovation and Sustainability, Global edition. 15th ed. Harlow, UK: Pearson Education Limited; 2018

[21] Ansoff HI, Kipley D, Lewis AO, Helm-Stevens R, Ansoff R. Implanting Strategic Management. 3rd ed. Springer Nature Switzerland: Palgrave Macmillan Cham; 2018. DOI: 10.1007/978-3-319-99599-1

[22] Hunger JD, Wheelen TL. Essentials of strategic management. 5th ed. New Jersey: Pearson Education, Inc; 2010

[23] Bass BM. Leadership and Performance Beyond Expectations. New York: Free Press; 1985

[24] Judge TA, Piccolo RF. Transformational and Transactional leadership: A meta-analytical test of their elative validity. Journal of Applied Psychology. 2004;**89**(5):755-768. DOI: 10.1037/0021-9010.89.5.755

[25] Burns JM. Leadership. New York: Harper & Row; 1978

Chapter 5

Management of Obstetrics and Intrapartum Emergencies

Amr Salem, Onyinye Allen Nwachukwu, Sabahat Zafar, Luis Yovera Leyva, Oana Velicu-Scraba and Venkata Sirisha Gurram

Abstract

Recent confidential enquires into maternal deaths in the UK have concluded that deaths due to obstetric hemorrhage have nearly doubled during the past triennium. The latest "Each baby Counts "Reported by Royal college of Obstetricians and Gynecologists has noted that approximately 76% of perinatal deaths and brain injuries could have been avoided by an alternative management. Lack of knowledge and human factors were the main contributory factors to poor outcomes. Substandard care is often due to "too little being done too late ", especially while managing emergencies during antepartum, intrapartum, and postpartum. All health care professionals including nurses should be familiar with management of emergencies with pregnancy.

Keywords: pregnancy, childbirth, maternal morbidity and mortality, maternal collapse, antepartum, intrapartum and postpartum bleeding, preeclampsia, septic shock, amniotic fluid embolism, breathless in pregnancy, convulsions and epilepsy in pregnancy

1. Introduction

Intrapartum emergencies are rare, but can be associated with significant maternal and fetal morbidity and mortality. It is important to know how to respond rapidly and appropriately. This chapter reviews selected issues and nursing care associated with emergencies in the intrapartum period, including cord prolapse, shoulder dystocia, amniotic fluid embolism (AFE), and hemorrhagic complications such as placental abruption, uterine rupture, vasa previa, and immediate postpartum hemorrhage (PPH). Simulation of potential obstetric emergencies is helpful to proactively assess systems, processes, communication, collaboration, and team member roles. If an obstetric emergency occurs, a debrief session is helpful to organize timing of event, management, and personnel involved. In addition, this discussion allows for all team members to discuss what went well and improvement opportunities.

2. Principles of resuscitation for 'maternal collapse' during pregnancy, labor and postpartum

Maternal Collapse is acute life threatening event in which the mother becomes unconscious due to cardiorespiratory or neurological compromise at any stage in pregnancy or up to 6 weeks postpartum.

The incidence of maternal collapse and sever maternal mortality is unknown. Recent studies estimate that maternal collapse occur in between 0.14 and 6 per 1000 births. In the hospital maternal collapse and sudden cardiac arrest are usually related to per partum events and the outcome depends on effective resuscitation and identification and effective treatment of underlining cause. Therefore staff on the hospital must be expertly trained in advanced life-support techniques and resuscitation equipment should be readily available.

During resuscitation, the mechanical ad physiological changes of pregnancy can have an impact on a successful outcome and should be considered.

Specific causes for maternal collapse.

While some underlying causes of maternal collapse are not preventable, it is important to note that maternal cardiac arrest occur frequently due to deterioration of underling critical illness. Care for women with significant pre-existing illness should therefore occur in a multidisciplinary sitting with place for pregnancy management and delivery. It is important to introduce a maternal early –warning chart for the observation of all pregnant patients in a hospital setting, to detect critical illness at the earliest possible stage [1, 2].

3. Most common causes of maternal collapse

3.1 Hemorrhage

Worldwide, Hemorrhage is still the leading cause of maternal mortality and it is the leading cause of maternal collapse on the delivery unit. The estimated incidence 3.7 per 1000 maternities. Predisposing factors are multiple pregnancy, high parity, placenta previa, uterine fibroids, and multiple previous caesarian sections, prolonged labour, maternal clotting disorders and preeclampsia. A high index of suspicion can be lifesaving. It is helpful to memorize the risk factors because hemorrhage can be concealed and pregnant women may lose a significant amount of blood without any hemodynamic disturbance. It is important to note that the blood loss is frequently underestimated and if hemodynamic changes become apparent, the mother has usually already lost third of her circulating blood volume.

3.2 Thromboembolism

A carful risk assessment for thrombotic complication should be performed in all pregnant women during the antenatal and postnatal periods. Multiple risk factors can make thromboprophylactic treatment necessary in pregnancy and postpartum for up to 6 weeks depending on risk assessment. Remember that deep venous thrombosis (DVT) of the pelvic venous system is often asymptomatic until pulmonary embolism develops.

3.3 Amniotic fluid embolism

The incidence of AFE is estimated at 1.25–12.5 in 100,000 maternities. While this is an unpreventable event, the speed of diagnosis determines the outcome. Survival rates have improved to 80%; however neurological morbidity is recognized. There is no diagnostic test to determine AFE; therefore, the clinical picture should lead to a high index of suspicion. Clinical features include respiratory distress, followed by cardiovascular collapse with hemorrhage due to coagulopathy within 30 minutes of delivery. AFE can also occur antepartum during labor and become manifest as fetal collapse of unknown origin that precedes maternal collapse. In all cases there is absence of any other significant medical condition or other explanation for the rapid deterioration.

3.4 Sepsis

Morbidity and mortality from pregnancy –related sepsis is common and has not significantly declined in recent years. Sepsis must be treated promptly as a medical emergency and appropriately managed with a 1 hour bundle to improve outcomes [3]. Obstetric risk factors include prolonged rupture of membranes, cervical cerculage, retained placenta and operative trauma. Patient related risk factors include obesity, anemia, diabetes mellitus, sickle cell disease and group B streptococcus infection. Adequate antibiotic prophylaxis for patients at risk is crucial. Common clinical signs are temperature, tachycardia and altered mental state, ranging from anxiety to confusion. Special attention should be paid to changes in the respiratory rate as an early diagnostic sign of the physiological reaction to a developing metabolic acidosis due to sepsis.

3.5 Complication of labor analgesia

Even in a correctly sited epidural catheter, a regular top up with local anesthetic drugs can cause maternal collapse due to hypotension; therefore regular blood pressure observations are required after each administration of local anesthetic.

3.6 Resuscitation 'S&T and ABC'

Preventing a cardiac arrest should be a key priority. Unstable women should be immediately positioned left lateral or left lateral tilted to prevent vena cava compression syndrome. Compromised venous return and reduced cardiac output can precipitate cardiac arrest in critically ill pregnant women. High flow oxygen should be administrated, and venous access established. Maternal hypotension (<100 mmHg systolic or < 80% baseline blood pressure reading) should be treated with a fluid bolus of crystalloid or colloid infusion. Reversible causes of maternal collapse should be considered and treated as necessary. Resuscitation efforts in pregnant women should follow the standardized A, B, C approach with no alternations in the basic algorithm or drugs. The following modification should occur to take into account physiological changes in pregnancy that may hinder successful resuscitation.

S&T: Shout for help and ensure a safe environment. Tilt the patient left lateral if visibly pregnant or beyond 20 weeks gestation. Use a wedge or ask another person to manually displace the uterus during resuscitation.

A for airway: Assess and open airway. Turn the patient onto her back (keep left lateral tilt or manually displace uterus). Check for airway obstruction. Use head tilt and chin lift. Secure airway with endotracheal tube as soon as possible or consider second generation supraglottic airway devices that can prevent aspiration. There is a higher incidence of failed intubation in pregnancy with significant maternal morbidity and mortality. Airway maneuvers should therefore be performed only by an experienced operator and ideally capnography used to confirm correct tube placement.

B for breathing: Assess breathing for 10 seconds. If the patient is not breathing normally start cardiopulmonary resuscitation (CPR).

C for circulation: check the carotid pulse and ensure volume replacement via two large-bore cannulas.

CPR Chest compressions should be performed slightly higher on the sternum than usual, as the maternal diaphragm is elevated in lateral stages of pregnancy. It is important to deliver efficient compressions, which can be less effective with a 15–30 tilt.

Venous access should be established above the diaphragm as soon as possible. Blood product including clotting factors should be made available at early stage of resuscitation.

Automated external defibrillator (AED): There is a small risk for inducing fetal arrhythmias with defibrillation; however, external defibrillation is considered safe in all stages of pregnancy [4].

4. Management of massive obstetric hemorrhage

Definition Blood loss >2000 mL (or > 30% of blood volume) is defined as massive obstetric hemorrhage (MOH). There is a tendency to underestimate rather than overestimate the actual blood loss.

Types MOH can occur either in the antepartum period secondary to placental abruption, placenta previa or accrete or in the postpartum period due to the '4Ts (tone, trauma, tissue and thrombin). Other rare obstetric disorders such as AFE or acute inversion of the uterus may also present with MOH.

Incidence PPH occurs in 2–10% of delivers but the incidence of major obstetric hemorrhage is estimated to be 3.7–5 per 1000 maternities.

It is estimated that every year about 356,000 women die during childbirth around the world. In the developing world the PPH occurs in about 4–10% of deliveries. The last report of the Confidential Enquires into Maternal Deaths in the UK has listed PPH as the third most common cause of maternal mortality [5]. Massive blood loss leads to sudden and rapid cardiovascular decompensation and coagulopathy.

4.1 Key etiological factors

Antepartum

- Placenta previa
- Placental abruption
- Rupture of undiagnosed secondary abdominal pregnancy
- Uterine rupture

- Morbidly adherent placenta (accrete, increate, percreta)

Intrapartum

- Amniotic fluid embolism (AFE) with coagulopathy
- Uterine rupture secondary to previous uterine scar or grand multiparty, especially with injudicious use oxytocin.
- Surgical compilations (extension of uterine angular tear during cesarean section)

4.2 Key points to massive obstetric hemorrhage

Visible Blood loss >2 L.

Ongoing bleeding (> 150 mL/min).

Loss of >30% of blood volume as assessed by visible blood loss (estimated blood loss or EBL expressed as percentage of estimated blood volume = EBL/100 mL/kg).

Rule of 30 (Rise of pulse >30/minutes, drop in systolic blood pressure by 30 mmHg, increased respiratory rate > 30 per minute, a drop in hematocrit [packed cell volume]by 30%), which is suggestive of at least 30% loss of blood volume.

Shock index (pulse rate/systolic blood pressure) 0.9. Normal Shock Index in pregnancy is between 0.7 and 0.9, as the pulse rate is less than systolic blood pressure.

Tense, tender abdomen with evidence of intrauterine death (massive placental abruption).

5. Management algorism HEMOSTASIS for postpartum hemorrhage

H Ask for Help and hands on uterus (uterine massage).

A Assess (ABC) and resuscitate (crystalloids 2 Colloids 1 L, oxygen by mask (15 L/min).

E Establish etiology (atonic, traumatic, coagulopathy or trauma) ensure availability of blood and administer ecbolic (drugs that contract the uterus: oxytocin or syntometrine intramuscularly).

M Massage uterus.

O Oxytocin infusion/ prostaglandins: IV/IM/per rectal (second-line medication to contract the uterus).

S shift to theater: aortic pressure or anti-shock garment/bimanual compression as appropriate.

T Tamponade balloon/uterine packing: after exclusion of tissue and trauma.

A Apply compression structure: B-Lynch/modified.

S Systematic pelvic devascularisation: uterine/ovarian/quadruple/internal iliac.

S Subtotal/total abdominal hysterectomy [6].

6. Complete the '3 E's' after every obstetric emergency

Examine- For heart rate, blood pressure, uterine contractility and vaginal bleeding and monitor urine output. Replenish lost fluid, blood and blood products adequately.

Explain the delivery event, possible reasons, complications and future plan of the care to the patient (i.e., debrief).

Escalate – complete the Incident Reporting Form and inform senior colleagues as well as to the team to identify learning points to continuously improve patient care.

7. Abdominal pain in pregnancy

Acute abdomen refers to abdominal pain of less than 1 week's duration requiring admission to hospital, which has not been previously treated or investigated.

Abdominal pain in pregnancy may be secondary to the anatomical and physiological changes of the pregnant state or may be totally unrelated to pregnancy.

Abdominal pain of any degree is a cause of significant maternal anxiety and constitutes a major reason for hospital attendance during pregnancy.

The gravid uterus enlarges to almost 20 times its normal 'non-pregnant 'size, which results in stretching of the supporting ligaments and muscles as well as pressure on the other intra-abdominal structures and layers of the anterior abdominal wall.

20% of the adnexal torsions occur or during pregnancy. This rarely includes torsion of the morphologically normal ovary.

8. Common causes of abdominal pain during pregnancy

8.1 Miscarriage

A combination between pain and vaginal bleeding should alert a clinician to a possible threatened, inevitable, incomplete or septic miscarriage. Pain is typically described as a 'cramping ach'. On examination, the fundal height of the uterus corresponds to the period of amenorrhea and signs of peritoneal irritation are absent. The internal cervical os might be opened or closed based on the type of miscarriage. An open os is diagnostic of an inevitable or incomplete miscarriage. Ultrasound examination is helpful to confirm viability, intra-uterine pregnancy and exclude a sub chorionic hematoma [7].

8.2 Ectopic pregnancy

Pregnancy is rarely located outside the normal endometrial cavity, most commonly in the fallopian tubes. Pain is typically unilateral and colicky. It may be superimposed on dull aching pain and may be associated with dizziness or fainting episodes. On clinical examination, unilateral iliac fossa tenderness, cervical excitation and adnexal tenderness may be elicited, The size (i.e., the measured fundal height) of the uterus is often less than what would be expected for the period of amenorrhea.

Demonestration of an empty uterine cavity on transvaginal ultrasound despite serum beta HCG levels of over 1500 IU/L may help clinician for the diagnosis.

Presence of any symptoms including abdominal pain or evidence of significant hemoperitoneum is a contraindication for medical treatment and surgical treatment is indicated. This includes emergency salpingectomy via laparoscopy or laparotomy.

8.3 Ovarian cyst accidents

Ovarian cyst complicate 1 in 1000 pregnancies and a vast majority are benign (98%). Pain is often described as intermittent and unilateral. Torsion also occurs more frequently on the right than the left, by a ratio of 3:2, owing to the presence of the colon on the left that limits the space available for torsion. Clinical examination may confirm tenderness in either iliac fossa and a large cyst may be palpable during abdominal and/or bimanual examination. However, in modern obstetric practice, the cyst is usually detected on ultrasound.

Most torsions and cyst accidents present as an acute abdomen and would warrant surgical treatment. Twenty percent of adnexal torsions occur during pregnancy. This also includes torsion o morphologically normal ovary. About 50% of cases of adnexal torsion have an associated ovarian mass.

In early pregnancy, symptomatic benign ovarian cysts may be removed by laparoscopic ovarian cystectomy. In view of inaccessibility of the adnexa in late pregnancy, a midline or Para median incision is recommended. Any ovarian cyst that exhibits sonographic features that are suggestive of malignancy should be referred to the oncological team for further imaging and appropriate treatment.

8.4 Placental abruption

Abruption placenta refers to the premature separation of normally situated placenta and it occurs in 0.5–1.5% of all pregnancies.

Abdominal pain may be present with or without vaginal bleeding. Fetal heart rate may be absent in sever abruption secondary to utero-placental insufficiency.

There may be varying degrees of hemodynamic compromise secondary to blood loss either vaginally or inside the uterus in the concealed variety.

Immediate senior input should be sought and management includes maternal resuscitation, correction of hypervolemia and coagulation abnormalities through a multidisciplinary approach. Emergency cesarean section should be performed in the event of suspected fetal compromise, once the woman is hemodynamically stable and her coagulation abnormality is corrected.

If an intrauterine death is confirmed, an amniotomy and oxytocin infusion may be commenced. Hemodynamic instability warrants immediate uterine evacuation to avoid morbidity and maternal mortality.

9. HELLP syndrome

Hemolysis, elevated liver enzymes and low platelets (HELLP) Syndrome often arises following preeclampsia. However, in 20% of the women, HELLP Syndrome may be the first presentation of preeclampsia. Women often present with acute right upper quadrant or epigastric pain. They may also have other preeclampsia stigmata that include headaches, vomiting, visual disturbances, irritability and altered consciousness. Systemic examination may reveal raised blood pressure. Abdominal examination might note epigastric pain or right upper quadrant tenderness. Investigation might depict hemolysis (raised lactate dehydrogenase >500 units/L; bilirubin >12 mg/L), raised liver enzymes (alanine transaminase >70 units/L) and low platelets. Management is aimed at stabilizing blood pressure, seizure prophylaxis, correction of any coagulation abnormality and delivery [8].

10. Conclusion

Obstetrics is a very high risk specialty associated with increased likelihood of patient safety incidents, mainly because this is the only specialty in which clinicians have to critically balance the interests of one human being (the mother) with that of another (the fetus), while providing care.

Rapid evolution of events during labour requires rapid decision-making skills in a highly pressured, high-risk environment, which may contribute to adverse incidents.

Maternity care involves multidisciplinary team approach involving midwives, obstetricians, neonatologists, anesthetists, hematologists, physicians, cardiologists, and other allied specialists Therefore, issues with communication, culture and team as well as task factors may contribute to patient safety incidents.

In obstetric practice, human factor play an important role in adverse events associated with cardiotocograph (CTG) interpretation and management of obstetric emergencies. Therefore, multiprofessional training in maternity care should incorporate human factors as an essential component.

Author details

Amr Salem[1*], Onyinye Allen Nwachukwu[2], Sabahat Zafar[2], Luis Yovera Leyva[3], Oana Velicu-Scraba[2] and Venkata Sirisha Gurram[4]

1 Basildon and Thurrock University Hospital, Basildon, Essex, UK

2 Southend University Hospital, Essex, UK

3 Broomfield Hospital, Chelmsford, UK

4 Basildon University Hospital, Essex, UK

*Address all correspondence to: amr.salem2@nhs.net

References

[1] Murphy CM, Murad K, Deane R, Byrne B, Geary M, McAuliffie FM. Sever maternal morbidity for 2004-2005 in three Dubline maternity hospitals. European Journal of Obstetrics & Gynecology and Reproductive Biology. 2009;**143**:34-37

[2] Dildy GA, Clark SL. Cadiac arrest during pregnancy. Obstetrics and Gynecology Clinics of North America. 1995;**22**:34-37

[3] Levy MM, Evans LE, Rhodes A. The surviving Sepsis Care Bundle: Update 2018. Intens Care Med. 2018;**44**(6):925-928

[4] Belfort MA, Saade GA, Foley MR, Phelan JP, Dildy GA. Critical Care Obstetrics. 5th ed. Oxford: Blackwell; 2010

[5] MBRRACE-UK. Saving Lives, Improving mother's Care: Surveillance of Maternal Deaths in the UK 2012-2014 and Lessons Learned to Inform Maternity Care from the UK and Ireland Confidential Enquirers into Maternal Deaths and Morbidity 2009-2014. UK: University of Oxford; 2014

[6] Royall College of Obstetricians and Gynecologists. Prevention and Management of Postpartum Hemorrhage. Green Top Guidelines No 52. London: RCOG; 2016

[7] Royall College of Obstetricians and Gynecologists. Management of Early Pregnancy Loss. Green Top Guidelines No 25. London: RCOG; 2006

[8] Chandraharan E, Arulkumaran S. Acute abdomen and abdominal pain in pregnancy. Obstetrics, Gynaecology and Reproductive Medicine. 2008;**18**(8): 205-212

Chapter 6

Are Hospitalized Patients Culturally Safe?

Parisa Bozorgzad

Abstract

My personal and professional experiences as a practitioner nurse, and a lecturer unveil that, in the present environment, patients, along with the fear of death and illness, face stressors such as being stranger to the treatment team, being unaware of the treatment process, fear of questioning, the unfamiliar environment of the hospital and its governing culture. In most cases, not only the values, beliefs and identities of patients are not taken into account in decision making, but also the atmosphere governing medical centers is somehow trying to instill their thoughts and beliefs in them. This makes decision-making solely on the basis of disease recognition, not pertaining to the patient's requirements. In such an atmosphere, the possibility of the patient's participation, cooperation and protection in daycare is threatened, and in many cases, it prevents follow-up and adherence to treatment and prevents us from the goal of improving the quality of patient-centered services with a view to clinical excellence. The concept of cultural safety, along with encouraging the practitioners to rethink, opens the way for the implementation and attainment of the ideals of emancipatory theory in nursing, which have been for years restricted to the scope of theoretical knowledge.

Keywords: cultural safety, patient-centered care, decision making, power imbalance

1. Introduction

The advent of modernity and its values into the philosophy of medicine had begun years before I became a nurse. In fact, I entered this major during the period of positivist revision. Yet, like many of my colleagues, I became a nurse with a positivist viewpoint. Fully confiding in western medicines, treatments and their effectiveness for all patients, I entered the hospital as an emergency ward nurse. However, the more I worked on patients, the more I noticed the differences between people and their disease impressionability. As a nurse, I was more focused on the patient himself and found that each patient perceives the disease in his own way. Accordingly, the burden and severity of the disease were different from patient to patient, but what caught my attention the most was their negative feelings about the experience of being hospitalized. Something more than illness seemed to bother them. I had heard them saying many times: "Do not see me falling on this bed, I was someone for myself." I do not know what was going on with them that they needed to remind us of their identity.

The turning point of all these thoughts was my hospitalization as a patient. I was admitted to the hospital where I worked. I had an independent identity there as a nurse, and I was in a friendly environment, so I thought it was the best place to get cured. But in a moment, after wearing the patients' uniform and with my first encounter with nurses, I lost all my identity. The illness had devoured not only my health but also my identity. Although familiar with all the concepts of care and treatment, I was not involved in treatment decisions. I was just a patient and only the doctors' and nurses' decisions were given to me. At the end of the first day of hospitalization, I was so full of negative and disturbing feelings that the disease was thoroughly forgotten. The health care provider's behaviors had a different story. They considered me someone who could not properly take care of herself and consequently got ill. While I was their colleague and knew all about the procedures and I was not afraid of them, I was blamed many times why I had not come earlier. I put myself in the shoes of patients who did not have my knowledge and realized what an unsafe and stressful place (hospital) they stepped in. Afterward, I reviewed that experience many times in my mind, and each time I felt the same sorrow. My feelings for myself as a nurse had changed.

With this concern and in search of a way to make the experience of hospitalization and illness lighter, I focused my studies on this area. Owing to my familiarity with philosophical concepts and philosophy of medicine, I realized how much I was entertained by the physiology of organism and body, and we are unaware of patients' cultural beliefs and values and their effects on determining the level of health and the type of people's experiences of health. Similarly, we have substituted the global standard treatment protocols for paying attention to patients' social status and cultural-historical and identity characteristics. The result is considering patients' identities based on their illness, such as epileptic patients or cancer patients. More painfully, the teachings are focused on the same principles [1].

However, in recent decades, the inefficiency of such an attitude has become more apparent and patients' dissatisfaction with the way services are provided, its coincidence with the customer-oriented issues and competition among medical centers has been an inauguration to criticize the biomedical model more than ever [2].

2. Cultural safety

Today, the emergence of new perspectives in the face of disease has fundamentally changed the meaning of treatment and care. In many developed countries, the patient is now considered among a set of factors determining the level of individual and social health, and the disease is considered not as a single phenomenon but as a product of the patient's Life-world [3]. In this case, Emami quotes Mardiros as saying, "When people look more deeply at their diseases, they realize that disease, illness and malnutrition are themselves symptoms of a deeper disease rooted in class differences, economic exploitation and political pressures" [4].

Nursing is no exception to these changes. Although holistic teachings were rooted in Florence Nightingale's point of view, and Madeleine Leininger was the first to formally emphasize the relationship between patient culture and nursing care [5], the integration of nursing with reductionist biomedical model and the desire to specialize in the care of various organs of the body caused the perspective of nursing to change at the same way as the philosophy of medicine changed. Perhaps the origin of these changes, coinciding with the introduction of the holistic paradigm, can be seen in the

1970s. Thus, health is defined as a feeling of well-being experienced and approved by the patient [6]. In fact, it is the patient's mental understanding that affects his or her satisfaction, and no one else but the patient himself can tell what matters to him [7].

Nowadays, the propagation of such attitudes has caused the patient to be seen with all his/her appurtenance and "culture" is considered as the framework of individual worldview and the factor shaping health behaviors [8]. Many international human rights treaties now recognize the "cultural right" as a principle based on respect for ethnic differences and acceptance devoid of judgment, and protecting these rights is the responsibility of health care providers' members, including nurses [9]. The International Council of Nurses (ICN) considers respect for human rights, including the cultural right, right to life, choice, human dignity and respectful behavior, which are not influenced by nationality, race, skin color, age and sex, as an integral part of nursing [10]. On the other hand, globalization and the expansion of communication, diversity and multiplicity of cultures and identities have changed the structure of societies. Now in many areas, therapists and patients do not share a common culture, and caring for patients with different cultures is a matter of course in 21st-century nursing [11].

In order to fulfill their mission of providing the community with health by communicating effectively with patients, all this has caused the health care providers to need a view beyond biological knowledge. My studies in this field eventually made me familiar with the concept of Cultural Safety. Regarding the issues raised, this concept emphasizes how the healthcare providers will be held responsible and accountable. In 1990, Irihapeti Ramsden introduced the concept of cultural safety as a result of colonialism and health inequalities in Maoris, which were among New Zealand's indigenous tribes [11]. New Zealand at that time was an independent country where, despite the end of the colonial era, the spirit of colonialism was still flowing in its interpersonal relationships, and this caused the country's largest indigenous minority to be in poor condition in terms of health and hygiene facilities. This concern was raised in 1988 by a group of Mao tribal nurses who relied on the concept of "safety" and found that regarding the prevailing culture of immigrant groups in the community there was no security for the natives in the Western biomedical educational space and this severely affected their health status [12]. They believed that despite the claims in today's society, care is not provided for individuals, but is planned for the groups or classes to which they belong, and because health care systems are influenced by the dominant culture and powerful groups of society and are planned according to their needs, there is no justice in this regard. On the other hand, health care providers are also trained to deal and communicate with the dominant groups of the society and recognize them as the "norm" [13]. Thus, cultural safety was born as a postcolonial concept. This concept is derived from clinical nursing, which focuses on the strength of nurses and other members of the health care providers to highlight the effects of power inequality on patients' health. Cultural safety is actually a radical concept that brings political perspective into the body of health knowledge and challenges "power" as a concept with the essence of politics in a knowledge-based context [14]. Given the effects of socio-political conditions on the attitudes and beliefs of the healthcare providers, especially nurses, this concept draws their attention to the impact of their views on patients' health [12].

Cultural safety means providing effective healthcare to a person with a different culture so that this care is approved by the individual and his family [15]. Emphasizing on "self-awareness," this concept challenges members of the healthcare providers in their intellectual background about the "power" [14], and creates a critical insight into the inherent power difference between the healthcare providers and the client, the therapist becomes aware of the impact of his or her thoughts on patients' health. In this regard, considering the patient's beliefs, values, personal experiences and cultural identity is inevitable [14, 16].

The word "culture" in cultural safety does not simply refer to ethnicity or race. Rather, in its broadest sense, it includes the age, sex, race, religion, social class, and economic and political status of individuals [17], this definition warns of the atmosphere of Racism and Ethnocentrism in health care providers and patient interactions. "Safety" is also derived from the idea of security in nursing and refers to the minimum standards that must be met to prevent harm to a person. Of course, along with physical safety standards, the role of moral standards is more prominent [18], and the patient's experience of illness shapes a sense of security or insecurity [19].

Cultural safety targets the therapist's attitudes and beliefs and emphasizes that the awareness of therapists about the impact of social, political and cultural factors on their thinking changes their viewpoints and is effective in creating safe interaction with patients [20]. According to this view, care is considered safe if the patient does not feel diminish, demean, disempowering [15] and if deprivation of health facilities and the social and political conditions of particular groups are recognized [21]. In other words, the patient's "identity" is not integrated into the disease and his/her individual needs are included in health planning [22]. Cultural safety is, in fact, the result of critics' efforts to achieve Emancipatory Theory. Hence, this concept can be considered as a facilitator for the transition from a purely empirical perspective to scientific intellect and wisdom. It is noteworthy that the Emancipatory Theory does not deny the importance of the empirical view, but it opposes its monopolism [23]. Therefore, cultural safety is not an emerging goal in nursing. Rather, it is a means of implementing what has been proposed in the theoretical realm for many years. In addition, this concept, along with encouraging the healthcare providers to rethink, paves the way for the implementation and achievement of the ideals of nursing emancipatory theories, which have not been outside the scope of theoretical knowledge for many years [24].

By creating a new attitude in the healthcare providers, cultural safety helps them to understand their truth and change their attitudes toward other ethnicities. In addition, cultural safety encourages the healthcare providers to be open-minded and do not blame the victims of socio-historical processes for what they are today and to be flexible with people who are different from them since the lack of security and fear of humiliation are among the factors that make patients refuse to go to medical centers on time. These feelings put the patient in a passive position against the culture that governs medical centers and threaten his/her cultural safety and this affects the health of a large segment of society [17]. Cultural safety aims to create an atmosphere free of threats and judgments for the patients [25].

In fact, cultural safety can be used as a tool to identify and analyze the relationship between the patient and the therapist.

When we look at therapeutic relationships through the cultural safety lens, we realize that the basis of the relationship between patients and therapists is the power of knowledge. This relationship is one-sided in nature and is surprisingly formed to meet the needs of therapists, like when taking a history, filling out forms or completing procedures. Although these activities are all aimed at doing the patient's work, they are imperative and the way they are done is as if the patient has to help the doctor to do her daily work. The healthcare providers and especially the doctors ask more questions. Choosing the topic of conversation, it's starting and finishing is

DOI: http://dx.doi.org/10.5772/intechopen.104511

determined by them, and patients are merely responders. In fact, the same concept of "low value conversation" of Mishler [26], prevails in medical centers: One question, one answer and then the next question. In fact, the relationship between the healthcare providers and the patients has become so classified and framed that even facing non-co-speaking patients is not a challenge for the healthcare providers, because the dominant language is the language that the healthcare providers speak. In this case, non-co-speaking patients cannot express their Life-world to the healthcare providers, so their attitudes, beliefs and desires are ignored. In this case, "language" comes out of the passive form of a set of words that express the meaning of the speaker and becomes a tool of strength or superiority of the healthcare providers. Because it is not possible to talk and bargain about what the patient wants and what the doctor deems appropriate, and these conditions lead to medical hegemony.

Cultural safety tells us that, in fact, patients do not consider the healthcare providers, especially physicians to be their servants due to their needs or even by habit. Rather, they see them in a higher and superior position and transfer the same view to the healthcare providers. Thus, a hegemonic relationship is formed in patient relationships and healthcare providers. The term "hegemony" was first coined by Antonio Francesco Gramsci (1937–1891) and implies the domination of a class not only economically but also in all social, political and ideological aspects. Hegemony is a form of control that is primarily exercised through the macro structures of a society [27].

In this regard, paying attention to the position of health services in today's world, Daniel Weber (2016) warns about the medicalization process of human societies and considers that it a product of medical hegemony (health care providers). He uses the term Medical Care Industry for this purpose. He believes that it is so due to the introduction of money and politics as two main factors symbolizing power in the medical field [28].

These conditions include the agency of the healthcare providers toward patients. This agency is present in all processes from diagnosis to treatment decisions. Accordingly, medical expression dominates the biological expression of patients because patients only answer doctors' questions and do not have the opportunity to express themselves, and this is the condition that cultural safety has been protesting against and warning about its formation in medical centers. Another issue that threatens patients' cultural safety is professional centrism. Claiming that the problems are specialized, the healthcare providers do not actually involve patients in making the decision. In many cases, they provide patients with information selectively. In other words, they convey to patients what they want (at their own discretion). I call this situation a "disease indemnity." This means that patients at the time of hospitalization should remunerate for their getting sick by abandoning their values, beliefs and preferences and accept the culture that governs the hospital [29] , cultural safety has passed through mere participation in the process of being ill and emphasizes "effective participation." The current situation in the field of patient participation is actually what cultural safety calls the product of colonialism and warns about it. In fact, the insistence of cultural safety on patient participation is ultimately the attainment of the right to self-determination [21] that the superior view of physicians, which is referred to as professional centrism, has practically negated. From a cultural safety perspective, the scientific superiority of the healthcare providers and specifically the physicians cannot be a valid reason for treatment decisions because these people do not know the patient's preferences. In fact, they make decisions for illness and not for the patient [25].

Specialism, on the other hand, draws a glass wall between the patient and the healthcare providers and divides them into two categories: "insider" and "other," in such a way that the "insider" is at the center, and "the other" is around. Thus, cultural colonization governing medical centers is not a suitable platform for the realization of cultural safety. The dominance of the biomedical paradigm in these centers leaves no room for attention to the individuality, culture and identity of the patient in the ideology of the healthcare providers. This bipolar view shifts the power toward the health care providers and does not allow the patient to express her/himself, and in such a case the patient is exposed to cultural risk and not cultural safety [29].

On the other hand, patients have an effective role in the formation of this culture. As Foucault recalls, this dominance has emerged with the patient's own complicity. It is clear that patients' perspectives are derived from the culture and social teachings. Today, the cultural institutions of society, of which the media is perhaps one of the most pervasive and effective ones, move to maintain and strengthen this dominance, willingly or unwillingly. Medicalization that Ivan Illich mentions [30] is widely advertised by the media. Making numerous medical programs and inviting medical staff to discuss and comment even on religious beliefs and rituals such as fasting, etc. contributes to accelerate this culture because people see all aspects of their lives from birth to death in their hands. In fact, influential organs in popular culture offer philosophies in which life is not possible without medical science, and in this way, they strengthen the hegemony of the healthcare providers.

Cultural safety can change totalitarian ideologies, and create critical insights into the members of the healthcare providers informing them the impact of their performance. Accordingly, while satisfying patients and promoting health services, it organizes and facilitates marginal movement to the center. As a converter tool to change the atmosphere of medical centers for the benefit of the patient, "cultural safety" can reduce the suffering of illness and hospitalization [14].

To achieve this goal, it is necessary for nurses and other members of the healthcare providers to have a view beyond the disease of the patient, and taking into account all the biological, psychological, social and cultural aspects to provide safe care that is approved by the patient. In the face of patients with chronic diseases, nurses and other members of the healthcare providers should pay special attention to the bio-world of the patient because these patients live with their disease and as a result, the disease can change the quality of their life for a long time. And this is exactly where understanding the patient's bio-world can be effective in providing safe services. In addition, it should be noted that without knowing the patient, safe and approved care cannot be provided. Therefore, a suitable bed must be provided to hear the patient and understand his expectations. Nurses and other members of the healthcare providers should be aware that standardizing treatment of patients not only means justice but also endangering their cultural security, creates conditions of inequality and the exercise of power.

Cultural safety is the result of a process that begins with cultural awareness and leads to cultural safety by understanding cultural sensitivity and cultural competence [22]. Cultural awareness means understanding the impact of culture on the formation of one's beliefs, values and political power and emphasizes that different cultures, subcultures and ethnicities have different values and views [31]. Cultural sensitivity means respecting and valuing different cultures. With such an attitude, one understands how culture affects one's personal and professional identity, and this is essential for establishing an effective cultural interaction [32]. Cultural competence is also understanding the values, beliefs and functions of patients' health that promote patients' health and is considered as an essential part of holistic care [31].

Thus, cultural safety is the product of a movement that begins with cultural awareness and eventually reaches cultural competence [33]. But, in many cases, the current education has remained at the level of cultural awareness. As a result, only existing cultural diversity is accepted, but the place of culture in the treatment of the disease and patients' views on the disease are not considered [14]. What is raised in cultural sensitivity is beyond mere recognition of differences.

According to this concept, even two people with a common culture can have different perceptions of the world [18], and understanding this can pave the way for cultural safety.

In other words, even in common contexts, nurses should not present care with their own pre-judgments and presuppositions, and this is the very emphasis on individualized care in nursing.

3. Conclusions

The healthcare providers behave as they are trained. What is taught in medical and nursing universities is the treatment of diseases based on the biomedical paradigm. This paradigm is knowledge-based and disease-oriented and does not take into account many individual and social factors. Therefore, a large group of factors affecting health is ignored. Neglecting things such as paying attention to individual and non-biological aspects of the disease causes inefficiency of the health system. Teaching these cases can make students be more effective people to maintain and promote health. Changing the viewpoints of nursing education custodians from the concept of "culture" is essential in this regard. It is necessary for nursing and other medical disciplines' students to learn that specialized knowledge does not necessarily outperform empirical knowledge, and treating the disease without knowing the patient's bio-world is just a mirage.

On the other hand, communicative inequality and information imbalance minimizes the possibility for the patient to participate in care procedure. Believing in supposed superiority due to their expertise, the healthcare providers unconsciously choose options that meet their own needs. The guided information neglects the patient's agency. In so doing, participation in treatment as a fundamental cornerstone in cooperation between the patients and curers is replaced by obeying treatment. This elite-oriented perspective contrasts sharply with a humanitarian and democratic process which is a necessity for a patient-curer relationship. In this case, the cure team identifies itself as an elite group with a consistent organization which considers patients as a formless mass being affected; thereby, the cure team feels superior and tends to convey such superiority to patients. In an atmosphere like this, the possibility for the patient to affect the care team is almost trivial or improbable, and this is a threat to the cultural safety of the hospitalized patients.

Acknowledgements

This chapter is a part of my research study and extensive studies conducted by me and my colleagues. Hereby, I express my heartiest gratitude to Professor Reza

Negarandeh, Professor Hamid Peyrovi, and Dr. AbouAli Vedadhir, who helped and guided me in performing the study.

Conflict of interest

The author declares no conflict of interest.

Author details

Parisa Bozorgzad
Nursing Care Research Center, School of Nursing and Midwifery, Iran University of Medical Science, Tehran, Iran

*Address all correspondence to: parisa.bozorgzad@gmail.com

References

[1] Matine P. Disease and Culture. Tehran, Iran: Farhameh; 2015

[2] Ping LLA. A conceptual analysis of nurses' customer-oriented behavior, job satisfaction and affective commitment in Malaysia. International Journal of Caring Sciences. 2015;**8**(3):774-782

[3] Al-Bannay H, Jarus T, Jongbloed L, Yazigi M, Dean E. Culture as a variable in health research: Perspectives and caveats. Health Promotion International. 2014;**29**(3):549-557

[4] Emami S, Pezeshki M. Holistic view in medicine. Iranian Journal of Medical Education. 2001;**1**(3):7-15

[5] Leininger MM. Leininger's theory of nursing: Cultural care diversity and universality. Nursing Science Quarterly. 1988;**1**(4):152-160

[6] Erickson H. Philosophy and theory of holism. Nursing Clinics of North America. 2007;**42**(2):139-163

[7] Ghods A, Vanaki Z, Kazemnejad A. Patients' satisfaction: Nurses' perspective. Iranian Journal of Medical Ethics and History of Medicine. 2010;**4**(1):47-61

[8] Ravindran N, Myers BJ. Cultural influences on perceptions of health, illness, and disability: A review and focus on autism. Journal of Child and Family Studies. 2012;**21**(2):311-319

[9] Johnstone M-J. Bioethics: A Nursing Perspective. New South Wales: Elsevier Health Sciences; 2019

[10] Oguisso T, Takashi MH, Freitas GF, Bonini BB, Silva TA. First international code of ethics for nurses. Texto & Contexto-Enfermagem. 18 Jul 2019;**28**. DOI: 10.1590/1980-265X-TCE-2018-0140

[11] Jeffreys M. Dynamics of diversity: Becoming better nurses through diversity awareness. Imprint. 2008;**55**(5):36-41

[12] Richardson S. Aoteaoroa/New Zealand nursing: From eugenics to cultural safety. Nursing Inquiry. 2004;**11**(1):35-42

[13] Woods M. Cultural safety and the socioethical nurse. Nursing Ethics. 2010;**17**(6):715-725

[14] Bozorgzad P, Raiesifar F, Poortaghi S. Cultural safety: A concept analysis. Holistic Nursing Practice. 2016;**30**(1):33-38

[15] Horrill T et al. Understanding access to healthcare among Indigenous peoples: A comparative analysis of biomedical and postcolonial perspectives. Nursing Inquiry. 2018;**25**(3):e12237

[16] DeSouza HR. Cultural safety: An overview. In: Lillie J, Larsen K, Kirkwood C, Brown JJ, editors. The Relationship Is the Project. Australia: Brow Books; 2020. p. 8

[17] Papps E, Ramsden I. Cultural safety in nursing: The New Zealand experience. International Journal for Quality in Health Care. 1996;**8**(5):491-497

[18] Curtis E et al. Why cultural safety rather than cultural competency is required to achieve health equity: A literature review and recommended definition. International Journal for Equity in Health. 2019;**18**(1):1-17

[19] Sooful P et al. Escape into culturally safe patient centered care. Noble

International Journal of Social Sciences Research. 2021;**6**(2):18-23

[20] Spector R, Cox L, Taua C. Cultural safety: Cultural considerations. Jarvis' Physical Examination and Health Assessment: ANZ Adaptation. 2012:40-60

[21] Bourque Bearskin RL. A critical lens on culture in nursing practice. Nursing Ethics. 2011;**18**(4):548-559

[22] Brascoupé S, Waters C. Cultural safety exploring the applicability of the concept of cultural safety to aboriginal health and community wellness. International Journal of Indigenous Health. 2009;**5**(2):6-41

[23] Bickford D. Postcolonial theory, nursing knowledge, and the development of emancipatory knowing. Advances in Nursing Science. 2014;**37**(3):213-223

[24] Ray MA, Turkel MC. Caring as emancipatory nursing praxis: The theory of relational caring complexity. Advances in Nursing Science. 2014;**37**(2): 132-146

[25] Bozorgzad P et al. A critical lens on patient decision-making: A cultural safety perspective. Nursing and Midwifery Studies. 2017;**6**(4):189-195

[26] Mishler EG. The Discourse of Medicine: Dialectics of Medical Interviews. Vol. 3. New Jersey: Greenwood Publishing Group; 1984

[27] Illich I. The medicalization of life. Journal of Medical Ethics. 1975;**1**(2):73-77

[28] Weber D. Medical hegemony. International Journal of Complementary Alternative Medicine. 2016;**3**(2):37-38

[29] Bozorgzad P, Peyrovi H, Vedadhir AB. Cultural Safety of Hospitalized Patients: A Critical Ethnography Study in School of Nursing and Midwifery. Teheran, Iran: Teheran University of Medical Sciences; 2017

[30] Van Deven T. The Native-English Teaching Program in Hong Kong. China: A Critical Ethnography; 2006. pp. 1-234

[31] Lin C-J, Lee C-K, Huang M-C. Cultural competence of healthcare providers: A systematic review of assessment instruments. Journal of Nursing Research. 2017;**25**(3):174-186

[32] Norton D, Marks-Maran D. Developing cultural sensitivity and awareness in nursing overseas. Nursing Standard. 2014;**28**(44):39-40

[33] DeSouza R. Wellness for all: The possibilities of cultural safety and cultural competence in New Zealand. Journal of Research in Nursing. 2008;**13**(2):125-135

Chapter 7

Somnambulism: Recent Findings

Sachi Sri Kantha

Abstract

Somnambulism is characterized as a parasomnia occurring during slow-wave sleep stages. It is also an autosomal dominant disorder, and its genetic locus has been identified at chromosome 20 q12-q13.12. The prevalence of somnambulism among children and adults has been estimated as 1–6%. Among the specific environmental factors precipitating somnambulistic episodes in adults, prescription drug use, alcohol, emotional stress, sleep deprivation, and certain psychiatric conditions have been suggested. Somnambulistic patients frequently cause injuries to themselves, family members who sleep nearby, and in-hospital settings to nurses who attend on them. Even cases of homicidal somnambulism have been reported. The lack of a suitable animal model to study somnambulism in controlled settings hinder appropriate pharmaceutical protocols to prevent this disorder among humans. Partial or total alleviation of somnambulistic symptoms in children and adults deserves the attention of health researchers.

Keywords: parasomnia, sleepwalking, treatment, trauma, violence

1. Introduction

In 1969, while introducing the electroencephalographic (EEG) recordings of sleep stages, Barbara Long [1] wrote, "We know that patients in hospitals, away from their usual sleeping environments and beset by the problems created by illness, frequently have difficulty meeting one of their most basic physiologic needs—the need for sleep—at a time when they require it most." In this commentary, Long briefly introduced insomnia as one of the health problems suffered by hospitalized patients. Subsequent reports by Williams [2] and Walsleben [3] passingly mentioned other sleep disorders, but failed to elaborate on somnambulism (in the lay term, sleepwalking).

In one of the anonymous early reports [4] that appeared on somnambulism in 1834, the recommendation offered for treating somnambulism was "*to seize the arms suddenly, and halloo in the ears until the sleep awake: of the application of a jug of cold water, by pouring it suddenly upon the head. In this latter case, however, care should be taken to have the body well rubbed with dry towels after the operation.*" Whether somnambulism will be permanently cured by this sort of crude treatment is open to doubt.

Nevertheless, medical knowledge on somnambulism, especially after the discovery of rapid eye movement (REM) sleep in 1953 [5] and the use of polysomnographic detection methods [6, 7], has accumulated in the past 65 years. Though it was widely believed until 1956, that somnambulism occurs during the dream phase (i.e., REM sleep stage), Jacobson et al. [8] demonstrated in nine subjects (seven men and two women, aged 9–23 years) that somnambulistic episodes occur during the N3 stage of slow-wave sleep (SWS) or non-rapid eye movement sleep (non-REM sleep). Specific electroencephalogram features of the N3 stage of SWS include delta waves (0.5–2 Hz, amplitude >75 μV) and slow oscillations (<1 Hz) [9]. For what is known about somnambulism until now, five reviews [9–13], with over 50 citations can be consulted profitably.

The objective of this chapter is to review recent developments on the presumed etiology, associated disorders, and treatment strategies currently available for somnambulism. The interdisciplinary relevance of somnambulism between medicine and law is also highlighted.

2. Etiology

Somnambulism or sleepwalking is one of the 15 parasomnias among the 81 recognized major sleep disorders. It is characterized by sudden arousal occurring at the SWS stages, resulting in walking behavior during a state of altered consciousness [14]. Somnambulism prevalence of 1–6% was indicated by Kleitman [15], "depending on whether the survey applied to the general public, hospital patients or to limited to children with sleep abnormalities." Thirty years later, Shapiro and Dement [16] offered a wider range (1–15%) of somnambulism prevalence, with children at the higher end of the range, relative to adults.

According to Kleitman [15], French physiologist Georges Henri Roger (1860–1946) had provided a good description of a typical sleepwalker, in his 1932 book *Les Troubles du Sommeil—Hypersomnies, Insomnies, parasomnies*. To paraphrase Kleitman [15],

> *"The sleeper performs various acts with a certain degree of dexterity and can avoid obstacles. But his behavior is characterized by a rigidity, which gives him the appearance of an automaton. He can answer questions correctly and is quite receptive to suggestions. He obediently carries out rather bizarre orders and tends to preserve attitudes passively imposed on him, exhibiting cataleptic properties. At the end of 15 to 30 minutes of activity, he goes back to bed, sometimes fully clothed, and wakes up next morning, quite surprised to find himself dressed. He can carry out dangerous tasks, like walking along the edge of a roof, which he would be afraid to do when awake" [15].*

Hereditary factors in the prevalence of somnambulism were first recorded in a short note, appearing in *Gazzetta degli Ospitali* 1930 by Clerici in a six-member Italian family (comprising of husband, cousin-wife, and their four children), all suffering from somnambulism. This fact was subsequently confirmed in other countries as well [6–7, 17].

Among a sample of 60 Caucasian subjects with somnambulism disorder, distributed in three countries (France, Switzerland, and Germany), Lecendreux et al. [18] reported that compared to eight (13.3%) age-matched controls, 21 (35%) somnambulists were positive for DQB1 allele of HLA-DQB antigen, and claimed this finding as a first genetic maker for somnambulism. HLA stands for human leukocyte antigen. Subsequently, Licis et al. [19] studied a four-generation Caucasian family in the USA consisting of 22 members, among whom nine were somnambulists and 13 were unaffected. Genome-wide linkage analysis from gathered DNA samples revealed the following facts—(1) genetic locus for somnambulism is present at chromosome 20q12-q13.12; (2) sleepwalking may be transmitted as an autosomal dominant trait with reduced penetrance;

(3) seven among the nine somnambulists were males; (4) adenosine deaminase gene (ADA) is the most likely candidate gene in the chromosome 20q12-q13.12 linkage interval due to its association with SWS during with somnambulism occurs.

Since 1956, polysomnographic studies in somnambulist patients have been conducted in the USA, Canada, and a few European countries [7, 8, 20–32]. A chronological compilation of significant polysomnographic studies is presented in **Table 1**. Two

Country	**Year**	**Somnambulists**			**Controls**			**Reference**
		Sample no.	Age (yr)		Sample no.	age (yr)		
			Range	**Mean ± SD**		**Range**	**Mean ± SD**	
USA	1956	34	n.r[1]		60	n.r[1]		Pierce and Lipcon [7]
USA	1965	9	9–23		Nil	—		Jacobson et al. [8]
UK	1990	5		28.4 ± 7.8	352	17–44		Crisp et al. [20]
USA	1991	8 [SW][2] 15 [SW + ST][3]	18–51		Nil	—		Hurwitz et al. [21]
Germany	1998	10		27.6 ± 3.4	n.r[1]		27 ± 3.7	Mayer et al. [22]
France	2000	3[SW][2] 2[SW+ST][3]	22–40	31.2 ± 2.2	11		32.1 ± 2.5	Espa et al. [23]
Switzerland	2000	1	16		Nil			Bassetti et al. [24]
Poland	2005	1	26		1	16		Szelenberger et al. [25]
Italy	2007	8	21–49		12		29.5 ± 8	Oliviero et al. [26]
Canada	2008	30	16–47		Nil	—		Zadra et al. [27]
France	2009	8 [SW][2] 30 [SW + ST][3]	11–72		25	'Age-matched'		Oudiette et al. [28]
Switzerland	2013	10		66 ± 11.6	Nil	—		Di Fabio et al. [29]
France	2014	12		27.4 ± 8.4	Nil	—		Perrault et al. [30]
Czech Rep	2015	52	19–63		20	20–57		Buskova et al. [31]
France	2017	89[SW][2] 80[SW without SS][4] 9[SW with SS][5]		29.2 ± 7.1 32.8 ± 10.4 32.5 ± 10.1	15	'Age-matched'		Dubessy et al. [32]

[1]*n.r = not reported, presumed to be in late teens to 20s, as the subjects were naval recruits and Electronics school students.*
[2]*Patients suffered from sleepwalking only.*
[3]*Patients suffered from both sleepwalking and sleep terror.*
[4]*Patients suffered from sleepwalking without sexsomnia.*
[5]*Patients suffered from sleepwalking and sexsomnia.*

Table 1.
Significant polysomnographic studies in somnambulist patients.

recognizable features revealed were, (1) Earlier studies, with two exceptions, did not have proper control groups; (2) Until 2015, the total number of somnambulist patients was less than 40. In the studies reported by Hurwitz et al. [21] and Oudiette et al. [28], the higher number of patients suffered from sleepwalking *and* sleep terror. The earliest study by Andre-Balisaux and Gonsette [6] in Belgium was omitted in **Table 1**, due to my lack of access in checking the complete text of the original paper.

Among the specific environmental factors precipitating somnambulistic episodes in adults, prescription medication use [33], alcohol [34], emotional stress [35], sleep deprivation [27], and certain psychiatric trauma [36] have been suggested. As such, a multifactorial etiology for somnambulistic disorder deserves recognition.

3. Associated disorders

Somnambulism-associated disorders/syndromes are presented in **Table 2**. These include alcoholism [34], brain tumor [37], bulimia [38, 39], epilepsy [40–43],

Somnambulism-associated Disorders/Syndromes	References
Alcoholism	Himemiya-Hakucho and Fujimiya [34]
Brain tumor	Prashad et al. [37]
Bulimia	Guirguis [38]
	Bell and Tomkinson [39]
Epilepsy	Pierce and Lipcon [40]
	Tinuper et al. [41]
	Cornejo-Sanchez et al. [42]
	Duffau et al. [43]
Hyperthyroidism	Ajlouni et al. [44]
Migraine	Barabas et al. [45]
	Giroud et al. [46]
	Pradalier et al. [47]
	Lopez et al. [48]
Nocturnal hypoglycaemia	Bell [49]
	Cebrian et al. [50]
Parkinson disease	Poryazova et al. [51]
	Di Fabio et al. [29]
	Oberholzer et al. [52]
Sexsomnia	Dubessy et al. [32]
Sleep-disordered breathing	Espa et al. [53]
	Guillaminault et al. [54]
	Guillaminault et al. [55]
Tourette's syndrome	Barabas et al. [56]
	Jimenez-Jimenez et al. [57]

Table 2.
Somnambulism associated disorders/syndromes.

hyperthyroidism [44], migraine [45–48], nocturnal hypoglycemia [49, 50], Parkinson's disease [29, 51, 52], sexsomnia [32], sleep-disordered breathing [53–55], and Tourette's syndrome [56, 57]. In a cross-sectional case–control study conducted in Montpellier, France, with 100 adult sleepwalkers (55 men and 45 women, aged 18–59 years), Lopez et al. [48] found 44% suffered from chronic pain, compared to 20% of controls. Those sleepwalkers with chronic pain were more likely to be older and had higher daytime sleepiness. As one of the limitations in this study, Lopez et al. [48] had noted that pain sensitivity was not measured. Di Fabio et al. [29] reported that 9% of their 417 Parkinson's disease patients were somnambulists, and concluded that sleepwalking in Parkinson's disease is associated with depression, higher disease severity, and higher functional disability.

4. Brain cortex volume in somnambulists

Compared to age and gender-matched control group, in 14 drug-free polysomnographically confirmed adult somnambulists (age range 21–39 years), an MRI study reported by Heidbreder et al. [58] showed significant decreases of gray matter in the left dorsal posterior cingulate cortex and posterior midcingulate cortex. The mean disease duration of adult somnambulists was reported as 19.2 ± 7.7 years (range 6–33 years). Though this finding is of interest, it remains to be replicated [59] in other sleep laboratories with children somnambulists as well. Whether children somnambulists also show similar significant gray matter decrease in the cingulate cortex areas deserves clarification. This is because, while the prevalence of somnambulism peaks in childhood, its percentage decreases in adulthood.

5. Treatment strategies: pharmacological and other treatments

No drug has been developed specifically to cure somnambulism [60]. However, based on case histories, clonazepam—a tranquilizer of benzodiazepine class patented in 1960, at 0.25–0.5 mg dose to be taken 1–2 h before sleeping [61–63], imipramine—a tricyclic antidepressant [64], paroxetine—a selective serotonin reuptake inhibitor [65] and ramelteon, a melatonin receptor agonist, at a dose of 4 mg/day [66] have been suggested for successful treatments. Though clonazepam has been the most widely used medication for non-REM sleep parasomnias with reported success, its use has been restricted in France, for the reason that it may increase sleep-disoriented breathing and induce sedation the following day [32].

In a recent review on medication-induced somnambulism, Stallman et al. [33] had identified 29 medications that are possible triggers for sleepwalking. For convenience, these medications have been categorized into five classes as follows—(1) benzodiazepine receptor agonists and other gamma-aminobutyric acid (GABA) modulators, (2) antidepressants and other serotonergic agents, (3) antipsychotics, (4) β-blockers, and (5) "others," including antibiotic ciprofloxacin.

Other types of treatments include hypnosis [67, 68], psychotherapy, aversive behavioral therapy [69], and the use of customized bed alarms. A recent review with 60 references by de Cock [70] is recommended for additional details on this theme.

6. Interdisciplinary relevance to medicine and law

While studying the records of 20 patients admitted to intensive care units, who had a diagnosis of self-injurious sleep behavior disorders, between 1982 and 1990, at the Minnesota Regional Sleep Disorders Center, USA, Schenck and Mahowald [62] recognized that three among the 20 suffered from chronic night terrors/sleepwalking abnormality. The influence of various stressors commonly found in the intensive care units (such as sleeping in an unfamiliar setting, sleep disruption/deprivation, medication administration/withdrawal, and psychologic distress) may aggravate the condition of sleepwalkers is one inference from this study. From a retrospective chart review study of patients older than 15 years, admitted to the emergency department at a university hospital in Berne, Switzerland, Sauter et al. [71] inferred that life-threatening injuries associated with somnambulism may occur. As such, when patients present with falls of unknown origin, the possibility of somnambulistic cause should be considered. The 11 trauma patients, Sauter et al. [71] encountered, had injuries identified as contused facial lacerations, head injury, contusion of ribs, cervical spinal dislocation, and paraplegia below the thoracic vertebral body.

Self-caused injuries [71, 72] not-withstanding, to a confused public, somnambulism seems to be a puzzling phenomenon that flirts between the boundaries of medicine and the law. The pros and cons of the rights and penalties for this class of sleep disorder patients who commit serious crimes, including homicides [73], during somnambulistic episodes, continue to be debated without any resolution [74–84]. A controversial issue is the use of somnambulism defense in cases involving alcohol-induced homicides. In reviewing the scientific evidence and forensic considerations, Pressman et al. [85] had inferred that a defense of alcohol-induced sleepwalking or confusional arousal becomes a very attractive legal strategy with the potential of acquittal for the defendant. This, despite the fact "there is no direct experimental evidence that alcohol predisposes or triggers sleepwalking or related disorders."

Quite a number of reports have appeared in the last three decades, implicating somnambulism with sexual misconduct as well [86–88]. Among the nine cases of sleep-related violence and nine cases of sexual behavior in sleep, published between 1980 and 2012, the sleepwalking defense was proposed in 11 among these 18 cases [89]. In their review of these 18 cases, Ingravallo et al. [89] indicated that the trial outcome was in favor of the defendant in 14 of 18 cases. As the forensic evaluations widely differed from case to case, they had concluded that "an international multidisciplinary consensus for the forensic evaluation of sleep-related violence and sexual behavior in sleep need to be developed as an urgent priority." Though clinical descriptions of somnambulists with sexsomnia as anecdotal case reports show an increase in this century [32], probably due to its titillating factor in the digital mass media, it is not easy to replicate somnambulist-sexsomnia episodes in hospitalized setting, except on unusual conditions that such patients have a bed sharer of the same sex or opposite sex, during the observation period.

7. Conclusions

As somnambulism has not been recorded in non-human primates, no animal model exists to study somnambulism under controlled settings for elucidation of its biochemical mechanism of origin [90]. As such, the available pharmacological treatments have to be considered as the scatter-shot approach of case studies without appropriate controls [91]. Thus, partial or total alleviation of somnambulistic symptoms in children and adults deserves the attention of health researchers. Adequately powered, well-designed clinical trials remain the need of the moment. The plea made by Chinthapalli [92], an associate editor of the *British Medical Journal*, that medical schools should consider sleep medicine education seriously in their curriculum also deserves recognition.

Conflict of interest

I declare no conflict of interest.

Notes

I became interested in the somnambulism phenomenon while serving as a Visiting Professor at Kyoto University, Primate Research Institute, Inuyama (Japan) and studying the activity-sleep behavior of New World and Old World Monkeys, between 2002 and 2006. I appreciate the discussions I have had with veterinarians, Dr. Kiyoaki Matsubayashi and Dr. Juri Suzuki, during that period.

Author details

Sachi Sri Kantha
MediPhone Inc., Minato-ku, Tokyo, Japan

*Address all correspondence to: sachisrikantha53@gmail.com

References

[1] Long B. Sleep. American Journal of Nursing. 1969;**69**(9):1896-1899

[2] Williams DH. Sleep and disease. American Journal of Nursing. 1971; **71**(12):2321-2324

[3] Walsleben J. Sleep disorders. American Journal of Nursing. 1982; **82**(6):936-940

[4] Anon. Somnambulism. Dublin Penny Journal. 1834;**2**:395-396

[5] Aserinsky E, Kleitman N. Regularly occurring periods of eye motility and concomitant phenomena, during sleep. Science. 1953;**118**:273-274

[6] Andre-Balisaux G, Gonsette R. Electroencephalography in somnambulism and its value for the establishment of an etiological diagnosis. Acta Neurologica et Psychiatrica Belgica. 1956;**56**:270-281 (in French)

[7] Pierce CM, Lipcon HH. Somnambulism: Electroencephalic studies and related findings. U.S. Armed Forces Medical Journal. 1956;7:1419-1426

[8] Jacobson A, Kales A, Lehmann D, Zweizig JR. Somnambulism: All night electroencephalographic studies. Science. 1965;**148**:975-977

[9] Zadra A, Desautels A, Petit MJ. Somnambulism: Clinical aspects and pathophysiological hypotheses. Lancet Neurology. 2013;**12**:285-294

[10] Berlin RM, Qayyum U. Sleepwalking: Diagnosis and treatment through the life cycle. Psychosomatics. 1986; **27**(11):755-760

[11] Fenwick P. Somnambulism and the law: A review. Behavioral Sciences & the Law. 1987;5(3):343-357

[12] Hughes JR. A review of sleepwalking (somnambulism): The enigma of neurophysiology and polysomnography with differential diagnosis of complex partial seizures. Epilepsy & Behavior. 2007;**11**:483-491

[13] Stallman HM, Kohler M. Prevalence of sleepwalking; a systemic review and metaanalysis. PLoS One. 2016;**11**(11):e0164769. DOI: 10.1371/journal.pone.014769

[14] Thorpy MJ. Classification of sleep disorders. Neurotherapeutics. 2012;**9**:687-701

[15] Kleitman N. Sleep and Wakefulness. revised enlarged ed. Chicago: University of Chicago Press; 1963. pp. 552

[16] Shapiro CM, Dement WC. Impact and epidemiology of sleep disorders. British Medical Journal. 1993;**306**:1604-1607

[17] Davis E, Hayes M, Kirman BH. Somnambulism. Lancet. 1942;**1**:186

[18] Lecendreux M, Bassetti C, Dauvilliers Y, Mayer G, Neidhart E, Taft LM. HLA and genetic susceptibility to sleepwalking. Molecular Psychiatry. 2003;**8**:114-117

[19] Licis AK, Desruisseau DM, Yamada KA, Duntley SP, Gurnett CA. Novel genetic findings in an extended family pedigree with sleepwalking. Neurology. 2011;**76**:49-52

[20] Crisp AH, Matthews BM, Oakley M, Crutchfield M. Sleepwalking, night terrors and consciousness. British Medical Journal. 1990;**300**:360-362

[21] Hurwitz TD, Mahowald MW, Schenck CH, Schluter JL, Bundlie SR.

A retrospective outcome study and review of hypnosis as treatment of adults with sleepwalking and sleep terror. Journal of Nervous and Mental Disease. 1991;**179**:228-233

[22] Mayer G, Neissner V, Schwarzmayr P, Meier-Ewert K. Sleep deprivation somnambulism. Effect on arousals, deep sleep and sleep stage change. Der Nervenarzt. 1998;**69**:495-501 (in German)

[23] Espa F, Ondze B, Deglise P, Billiard M, Besset A. Sleep architecture, slow wave activity and sleep spindles in adult patients with sleepwalking and sleep terrors. Clinical Neurophysiology. 2000;**111**:929-939

[24] Bassetti C, Vella S, Donati F, Wielepp WB. SPECT during sleepwalking. Lancet. 2000;**356**:484-485

[25] Szelenberger W, Niemcewicz S, Dabrowska AJ. Sleepwalking and night terrors: Pychopathological and psychophysiological correlates. International Review of Psychiatry. 2005;**17**(4):263-270

[26] Oliviero A, Della Marca G, Tonali PA, Pilato F, Saturno E, Dileone M, et al. Functional involvement of central cortex in adult sleepwalking. Journal of Neurology. 2007;**254**:1066-1072

[27] Zadra A, Pilon M, Montplaisir J. Polysomnographic diagnosis of sleepwalking: Effects of sleep deprivation. Annals of Neurology. 2008;**63**:51-519

[28] Oudiette D, Leu S, Pottier M, Buzare MA, Brion A, Arnulf I. Dreamlike mentations during sleepwalking and sleep terrors in adults. Sleep. 2009;**32**(12):1621-1627

[29] Di Fabio N, Poryazova R, Oberholzer M, Baumann CR, Bassetti CL. Sleepwalking, REM sleep behavior disorder and overlap parasomnia in patients with Parkinson's disease. European Neurology. 2013;**70**:297-303

[30] Perrault R, Carrier J, Desautels A, Montplaisir J, Zadra A. Electroencephalographic slow waves prior to sleepwalking episodes. Sleep Medicine. 2014;**15**:1468-1472

[31] Buskova J, Pisko J, Pastorek L, Sonka K. The course and character of sleepwalking in adulthood: A clinical and polysomnographic study. Behavioral Sleep Medicine. 2015;**13**:169-177

[32] Dubessy AL, Leu-Semenescu S, Attali V, Maranci JB, Arnulf I. Sexsomnia: A specialized non-REM parasomnia? Sleep. 2017;**40**(2):1-9

[33] Stallman HM, Kohler M, White J. Medication induced sleepwalking: A systematic review. Sleep Medicine Reviews. 2018;**37**:105-113

[34] Himemiya-Hakucho A, Fujimiya T. An unusual case of drunk driving in Japan: Alcohol-related sleepwalking. Acta Medica Okayama. 2021;**75**(2):255-259

[35] Crisp AH. The sleepwalking/night terrors syndrome in adults. Postgraduate Medical Journal. 1996;**72**:599-604

[36] Culogeras RC. Sleepwalking and the traumatic experience. International Journal of Psychoanalysis. 1982;**63**:483-489

[37] Prashad PS, Marcus CL, Brown LW, Dlugos DJ, Feygin T, Harding BN, et al. Brain tumor presenting as somnambulism in an adolescent. Pediatric Neurology. 2013;**49**:209-212

[38] Guirguis W. Sleepwalking as a symptom of builimia. British Medical Journal. 1986;**293**:587-588

[39] Bell JA, Tomkinson JS. Sleepwalking as a symptom of bulimia. British Medical Journal. 1986;**293**:1239

[40] Pierce CM, Lipcon HH. Clinical relationship of enuresis to sleep walking and epilepsy. AMA Archives of Neurology & Psychiatry. 1956;**76**:310-316

[41] Tinuper P, Provini F, Bisulli F, Lugaresi E. Hyperkinetic manifestations in nocturnal frontal lobe epilepsy, semeiological featuresand physiopathological hypothesis. Neurological Science. 2005;**26**:s210-s214

[42] Cornejo-Sanchez DM, Carrizosa-Moog J, Cabrera-Hemer D, Solarte-Mila R, Gomez-Castillo C, Thomas R, et al. Sleepwalking and sleep paralysis: Prevalence in Colombian families with genetic generalized epilepsy. Journal of Child Neurology. 2019;**34**(9):491-498

[43] Duffau H, Kujan M, Tailandier L. Episodic nocturnal wandering in a patient with epilepsy due to aright temporopinsular low-grade glioma: Relief following resection. Journal of Neurosurgery. 2006;**104**:436-439

[44] Ajlouni KM, Ahmad AT, Al-Zahiri MM, Ammari FL, Jarrah NS, Abujbara MA, et al. Sleepwalking associated with hyperthyroidism. Endocrine Practice. 2005;**11**(1) :5-10

[45] Barabas G, Ferrari M, Matthews WS. Childhood migraine and somnambulism. Neurology. 1983;**33**:948-949

[46] Giroud M, d'Athis P, Guard O, Dumas R. Migraine somnambulism: A survey of 122 migraine patients. Revue Neurologique. 1986;**142**:42-46

[47] Pradalier A, Giroud M, Dry J. Somnambulism, migraine and propranolol. Headache. 1987;**27**(3):143-145

[48] Lopez R, Jaussent I, Dauvilliers Y. Pain in sleepwalking: A clinical enigma. Sleep. 2015;**38**(11):1693-1698

[49] Bell DSH. Nocturnal hypoglycaemia presenting as somnambulism. Diabetologia. 2010;**53**:2066-2067

[50] Cebrian S, Gimeno O, Orozco D, Pertusa S. Hypoglycaemia and somnambulism: A case report. Diabetes & Metabolism. 2012;**38**:574-575

[51] Poryazova R, Waldvogel D, Bassetti CL. Sleepwalking in patients with Parkinson disease. Archives in Neurology. 2007;**64**(10):1524-1527

[52] Oberholzer M, Poryazova R, Bassetti CL. Sleepwalking in Parkinson's Diesease: A questionnaire-based survey. Journal of Neurology. 2011;**258**:1261-1267

[53] Espa F, Dauvilliers Y, Ondze B, Billiard M, Besset A. Arousal reactions in sleepwalking and night terrors in adults: The role of respiratory events. Sleep. 2002;**25**:871-875

[54] Guilleminault C, Palombini L, Pelayo R, Chervin RD. Sleepwalking and sleep terrors in prepubertal children: What triggers them. Pediatrics. 2003;**111**:17-25

[55] Guilleminault C, Lee JH, Chan A, Lopez MC, Huang YS, da Rosa A. A non-REM-sleep instability in recurrent sleepwalking in prepubertal children. Sleep Medicine. 2005;**6**:515-521

[56] Barabas G, Matthews WS, Ferrari M. Somnambulism in children with Tourette syndrome. Developmental Medicine and Child Neurology. 1984;**26**:457-460

[57] Jimenez-Jimenez Flonso-Navarro H, Garcia-Martin E, Agundez JAG. Sleep

disorders in Tourette syndrome. Sleep Medicine Reviews. 2020;**53**:101335. DOI: 10.1016/j.smrv.2020.101335

[58] Heidbreder A, Stefani A, Brandauer E, Steiger R, Kremser C, Gizewski E, et al. Gray matter abnormalities of the dorsal posterior cingulate in sleepwalking. Sleep Medicine. 2017;**36**:152-155

[59] Pressman MR. The neurophysiological and neurochemical effects of alcohol on the brain are inconsistent with current evidence based models of sleepwalking. Sleep Medicine Reviews. 2019;**43**:92-95

[60] Arnulf I. Sleepwalking. Current Biology. 2018;**28**:R1283-R1295

[61] Kavey NB, Whyte J, Resor SR, Gidro-Frank S. Somnambulism in adults. Neurology. 1990;**40**(5):749-752

[62] Schenck CH, Mahowald MW. Injurious sleep behavior disorders (parasomnias) affecting patients on intensive care units. Intensive Care Medicine. 1991;**17**:219-224

[63] Anon. Drugwatch. American Journal of Nursing. 1996;**96**(10):60

[64] Cooper AJ. Treatment of coexistent night-terrors and somnambulism in adults with imipramine and diazepam. Journal of Clinical Psychiatry. 1987;**48**:209-210

[65] Lillywhite AR, Wilson SJ, Nutt DJ. Successful treatment of night terrors and somnambulism with paroxetine. British Journal of Psychiatry. 1994;**164**:551-554

[66] Sasayama D. Effective treatment of night errors and sleepwalking with Ramelteon. Journal of Child and Adolescent Psychopharmacology. 2016;**26**(10):948

[67] Eliseo TS. The hypnotic treatment of sleepwalking in an adult. American Journal of Clinical Hypnosis. 1975; **17**(4):272-276

[68] Stallman HM, Kohler M. A systematic review of treatments for sleepwalking: 100 years of case studies. Sleep and Hypnosis. 2017;**19**(2):21-29

[69] Mayer RG. A behavioral treatment of sleepwalking associated with test anxiety. Journal of Behavior Therapy and Experimental Psychiatry. 1975;**6**(2):167-168

[70] De Cock VC. Sleepwalking. Current Treatment Options in Neurology. 2016;**18**:6. DOI: 10.1007/s11940-015-0388-8

[71] Sauter TC, Veerakatty S, Haider DG, Geiser T, Ricklin ME, Exadaktylos AK. Somnambulism: Emergency department admissions due to sleepwalking-related trauma. Western Journal of Emergency Medicine. 2016;**17**(6):709-712

[72] Szabo J, Vida Z. Fracture of the leg while sleeping: Drug-induced somnambulism in adulthood. Sleep and Vigilance. 2020;**4**:43-45

[73] Bonkalo A. Impulsive acts and confusional states during incomplete arousal from sleep: Criminological and forensic implications. Psychiatric Quarterly. 1974;**48**:400-409

[74] Legal correspondent. Sleepwalking and guilt. British Medical Journal. 1970;**2**:186

[75] Broughton R, Billings R, Cartwright R, Doucette D, Edmeads J, Edwardh M, et al. Homicidal somnambulism: A case report. Sleep. 1994;**17**(3):253-264

[76] Broughton RJ, Shimizu T. Sleep related violence: A medical and forensic challenge. Sleep. 1995;**18**(9):727-730

[77] Cartwright R. Sleepwalking violence: A sleep disorder, a legal dilemma and a psychological challenge. American Journal of Psychiatry. 2004;**161**:1149-1158

[78] Horn M. A rude awakening; what to do with the sleepwalking defense? Boston College Law Review. 2004;**46**(1):149-182

[79] Xu MZ. Sexsomnia: A valid defense to sexual assault? Journal of Gender, Race and Justice. 2009;**12**(3):687-712

[80] Weiss KJ, Watson C, Markov D, Del Busto E, Foubister N, Doghramji K. Parasomnias, violence and the law. Journal of Psychiatry & Law. 2011;**39**(2):249-286

[81] Siclari F, Tononi G, Bassetti C. Death by sleepwalker. Scientific American Mind. 2012;**23**(3):38-41

[82] Popat S, Winslade W. While you were sleepwalking: Science and neurobiology of sleep disorders & the enigma of legal responsibility of violence during parasomnia. Neuroethics. 2015;**8**:203-214

[83] Stallman HM. Sleepwalking as a defence for illegal behavior: A commentary on Popat & Winslade. Neuroethics. 2015;**8**:335-337

[84] Sio D, Di Nucci E. Pushing the margins of responsibility: Lessons from Park's somnambulistic killing. Neuroethics. 2018;**11**:35-46

[85] Pressman MR, Mahowald MW, Schlenck CH, Bornemann MC. Alcohol-induced sleepwalking or confusional arousal as a defense to criminal behavior: A review of scientific evidence, methods and forensic considerations. Journal of Sleep Research. 2007;**16**:198-212

[86] Buchanan A. Sleepwalking and indecent exposure. Medicine Science and the Law. 1991;**31**(1):38-40

[87] Schenck CH, Mahowald MW. An analysis of a recent criminal trial involving sexual misconduct with a child, alcohol abuse and a successful sleepwalking defence: Arguments supporting two proposed new forensic categories. Medicine Science and the Law. 1991;**38**(2):147-152

[88] Mohanty K. Transmission of chlamydia and genital warts during sleepwalking. International Journal of STD & AIDS. 2008;**19**(2):129-130

[89] Ingravallo F, Poli F, Gilmore EV, Pizza F, Vignatelli L, Schenk CH, et al. Sleep-related violence and sexual behavior in sleep: A systematic review of medical-legal case reports. Journal of Clinical Sleep Medicine. 2014;**10**(8):927-935B

[90] Kantha SS. Is somnambulism a distinct disorder of humans and not seen in non-human primates? Medical Hypotheses. 2003;**61**:517-518

[91] Harris M, Grunstein RR. Treatments for somnambulism in adults: Assessing the evidence. Sleep Medicine Reviews. 2009;**13**:295-297

[92] Chinthapalli K. We need to wake up to the value of sleep medicine. British Medical Journal. 2014;**349**:g6099. DOI: 10.1136/bmj.g6099

Chapter 8

Lautenbach Irrigation System

Princess Busisiwe Siphiwe Mbatha

Abstract

Osteomyelitis is infection of bone and frequently seeds in trabecular areas affecting both bone and bone marrow. Bone infection differs from soft-tissue infection since bone consists of a collection of rigid compartments. Bone is thus more susceptible than soft tissues to vascular damage and cell death due to pressure in acute inflammation. Unless it is rapidly suppressed, bone infection will inevitably lead to necrosis. Chronic infection is seldom eradicated by antibiotics alone. Yet bactericidal drugs are important to suppress the infection and prevent its spread to healthy bone and to control acute flares. The choice of antibiotic depends on microbiological studies, but the drug must be capable of penetrating sclerotic bone and should be non-toxic with long-term use. A different technique is the Lautenbach approach, involving radical excision of all avascular and infected tissue followed by closed irrigation and suction drainage, and an appropriate antibiotic solution in high concentration to allow the 'dead space' to be filled by vascular granulation tissue.

Keywords: infection, chronic osteomyelitis, Lautenbach irrigation system, D.R.I, antibiotics

1. Introduction

The Lautenbach procedure involves debridement, intramedullary reaming and the insertion of double-lumen tubes to establish both a local antibiotic delivery system and cavity analysis for volume and culture (**Figure 1**). The end-point of treatment is when the irrigate produces three consecutive clear cultures with improvement in the blood indices and obliteration of the cavity volume [1–3].

In theater, the patient's affected limb is debrided, and sequestra are removed and cleaned. After that holes will be made (Reaming) on the bone. These holes will be enough to insert an irrigation tube, which is a double-lumen tube that means the tube has a smaller tube inside. There is one big tube (perforated) which drains the irrigation fluid from the patient and an intra-catheter inside that administers an antibiotic to the bone and its bone marrow. These tubes will stay with the patient from two weeks upwards or until the patient is cleared of infection.

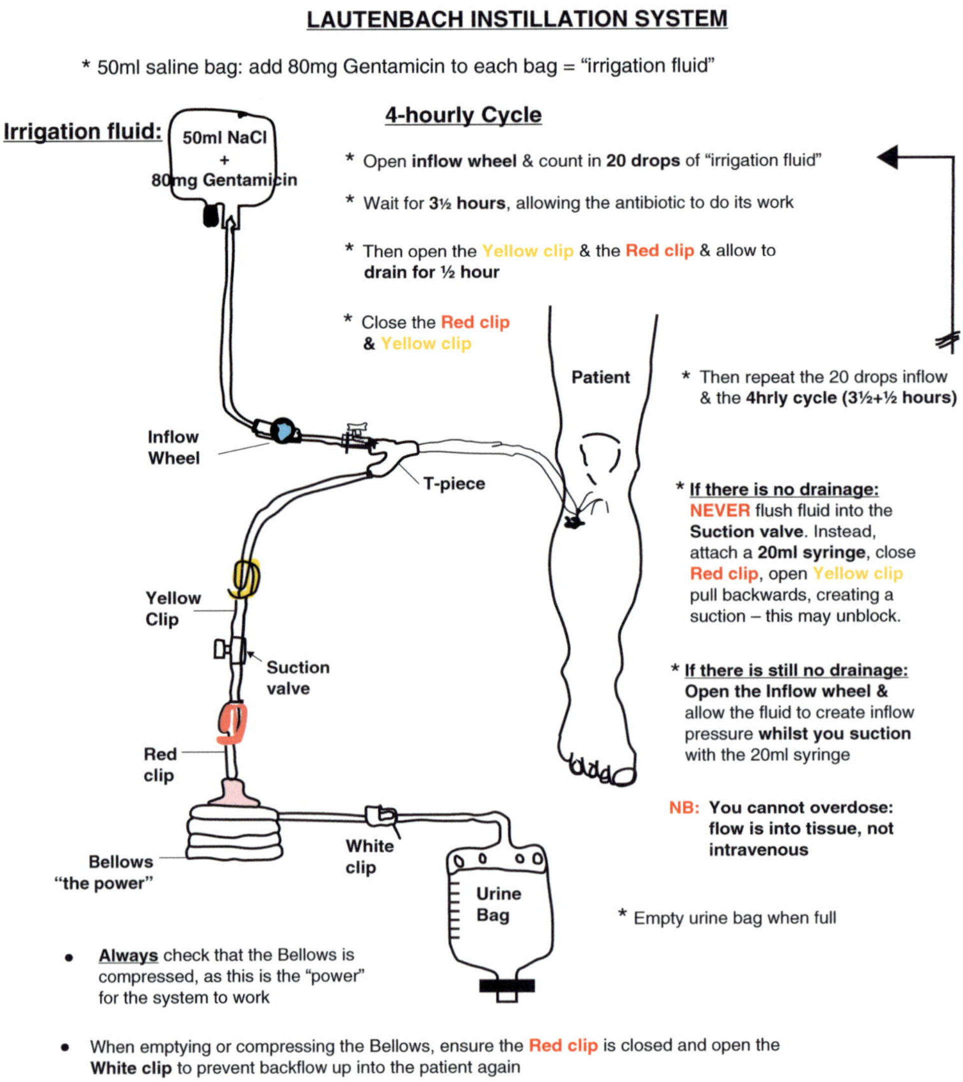

Figure 1.
Diagram of the Lautenbach irrigation system. Author: Charlotte Maxeke, Ward 369, Johannesburg Academic Hospital, South Africa. Adapted from original drawing, used with permission.

2. Irrigation system contents

- An administration set that almost looks like an intravenous infusion line to which is attached to a 50 ml antibiotic bag. This line which carries the antibiotic connects to the perforated tube through a Y-connection and the same administration set connects to a three-way stopcock and it delivers the antibiotic through the intra-catheter (a smaller tube that goes inside the bigger tube)
- A bellow that looks like a portovac drain but cannot be opened to maintain continuous negative suction.

- A drainage bag that looks like a urine bag but it has a tube permanently connected to the bellow.

3. Nursing management

On arrival in the ward from the recovery room, the nurse in charge of a patient post insertion of the Lautenbach irrigation system should do the following:-.

Postoperative vital data monitoring must be done as per hospital protocol. This includes checking of temperature, pulse, respiration, blood pressure, and oxygen saturation, which should be between 94 and 100% on room air. If the patient desaturates; 40% oxygen via face mask should be administered and the orthopedic surgeon on call should be informed to do arterial blood gases and also to take blood for post-operative full blood count and urea and electrolyte. As this is a major orthopedic procedure these patients bleed a lot and might need an intra-operative blood transfusion or postoperative blood transfusion depending on the condition of the patient. The patient may come back from the theatre with one, two, or even three irrigation tubes. These should be labeled, especially if there is more than one irrigation tube as follows; proximal tube, medial tube, and distal tube or tube 1, tube 2, and tube 3. The tube closest to the midline of the body of the patient would be labeled as a proximal tube and the tube that is situated further away from the body is labeled distal tube or tube 3 respectively.

The operated site should be checked as soon as possible so that the patient can be dressed with a pressure bandage to contain the bleeding. Whilst repacking the dressing; another nurse should open the red and yellow clips and let the irrigations drain regardless of time. This means for example; if the patient came back from the theater at around 16 h05 the drains should be drained from approximately 16 h10 till 18 h00, whilst monitoring the drainage. If the drainage is above 250 ml post operatively the irrigation system; (both yellow and red clips) should be closed and the orthopedic surgeon should be informed. That much drainage is concerning.

The gold standard antibiotic that is used postoperatively is gentamicin 80 mg in 50 ml of sodium chloride 0.9%. Sometimes in theater, the nursing staff will add 320 mg of gentamicin in 200 ml of sodium chloride 0.9%. This is not totally wrong but it is not ideal in a ward situation. This should be changed from 80 mg to 50 ml of sodium chloride 0.9% as soon as the patient is stabilized in the ward. Gentamicin mixed with sodium chloride will only last for two days at room temperature. So mixing 320 mg with 200 ml of saline is actually wasteful in nature and might as well prolong the patient's hospital stay because what if it is not changed at due time because 200 ml is seemingly enough to run for a few weeks.

Check for any leakage or oozing from the wound site. Do not remove dressings from the theater if oozing is noted. Dressings from the theater will only be removed on the day of removal of the irrigation system as a whole. Apply orthopedic wool and crepe bandage and monitor bleeding. In an ideal situation there should not be any bleeding at all, more often than not the report from the surgeon post operatively would be a space was left on the wound for various reasons [4], that would make exudate escape from the tubes to the dressing itself.

4. Protocol for irrigation maintenance

This is a very easy procedure to do as it is repeated every four hours. Even a patient can be taught how to do it without any issues. The disadvantage to this is that the

09H30-10H00	Open yellow clip and red clip. Let it drain for thirty minutes.
10H00	Close yellow clip and red clip. Administer 20 drops of an antibiotic.
13H30-14H00	Open yellow and red clip. Let it drain for thirty minutes.
14H00	Close yellow clip and red clip. Administer 20 drops of an antibiotic.
17H30-18H00	Open yellow and red clip. Let it drain for thirty minutes.
18H00	Close yellow clip and red clip. Administer 20 drops of an antibiotic.
21H30-22H00	Open yellow and red clip. Let it drain for thirty minutes.
22H00	Close yellow clip and red clip. Administer 20 drops of an antibiotic.
01H30-02H00	Open yellow and red clip. Let it drain for thirty minutes.
02H00	Close yellow clip and red clip. Administer 20 drops of an antibiotic.

These yellow, red, blue, or white clips are also called pinch clamps.

patients are often in a hurry to get discharged and they would assume that administering more than 20 drops of antibiotics at a go will help them get better sooner than expected, which is never the case. They will be overdosing on the tissues. Instead; the irrigation system will start leaking from the wound site.

5. Specimen collection

The specimens are collected three times a week, that is, Mondays, Wednesdays and Fridays [4]. Before collecting a specimen, the nurse responsible for the patient should prepare a trolley. Aseptic technique should be maintained at all times to avoid contaminating the specimen. The trolley should be cleaned with a disinfectant using an S shape. A sterile green cloth should be put on top of the trolley. Two 20 ml sterile syringes should be opened from their packaging and thrown on the sterile cloth. A packet of sterile gloves should also be put on the sterile cloth. An alcohol swab should be put on the bottom of the trolley with specimen bottle. If the alcohol swabs are not available, sterile cotton wool swabs drenched in a disinfectant should be used. A nurse who is taking a specimen should have another nurse who will open an alcohol swab for her, so sterile cotton swabs are better if there is no one to open the readymade alcohol swabs.

The nurse must then wash her hands and don gloves. After wearing gloves, would look for the port (Also called suction valve) between the yellow and red pinch clamp. This port should be cleaned thoroughly with an alcohol swab before opening it. The nurse must remove the cap connect the 20 ml syringe and then open the yellow pinch clamp. The red pinch clamp must not be touched at all during the collection of the specimen. The nurse must withdraw the first specimen and close the yellow pinch clamp. That specimen must be discarded and a second 20 ml syringe must be connected to the port so as to get a fresh new specimen directly from the wound site. The first specimen must have been sitting there in the tube for a long time and it might give a wrong result, also; using two syringes assists in unblocking of the irrigation system if this is the case . Once enough specimen is collected the yellow pinch clamp must be closed and the port must be closed. It is advisable to clean the cap with the disinfectant before putting it back on the port.

If the patient has more than one tube the same procedure should be repeated on another tube making sure that new gloves and syringes are used. The specimens should be labeled accordingly. The laboratory form should be filled with a patient's name, hospital number, doctor who is in charge of the patient's details, ward number, date and time the specimen was collected, and the diagnosis of the patient. The wound site should also be included in the laboratory form, for example, the right tibia, left humerus, right femur, etc. The specimen type should be marked as Irrigation Fluid, not blood even though it looks like blood a few days postoperatively. The investigation required should be indicated as Microscopy/Culture/Sensitivity in the laboratory form. After that, the specimen should be sent to the laboratory and it would take 24 to 48 hours for the results to come out, depending on the laboratory. If the patient has more than one irrigation tube, a separate laboratory form should be used for each specimen collected on each tube.

A nurse should make a note on the progress notes for doctors that a specimen has been collected. A lab sticker with a reference number for the laboratory should be stuck underneath the signature of the nurse who took the specimen so that it becomes easier for the medical personnel to trace the results for the patient.

Once results are received by the ward a professional nurse can read them and act accordingly. For example, if the patient cultured Staphylococcus Aureas, which is sensitive to Cloxacillin the professional nurse should put 1 g of cloxacillin in 50 ml sodium chloride and remove the one that has gentamycin in it. The doctor should be made aware of this development but there is no need to wait for further instructions to change antibiotics as the protocol allows the nursing staff to do so. Precaution should be taken with penicillin drugs and the patient's allergy should be considered. If the patient has MRSA the irrigations should be changed to vancomycin and the patient should be isolated in a private room or placed next to a window in hospitals where there are no isolation rooms. Universal precautions should be abided by at all times. With patients who have cultured MRSA, the surgeon would prescribe vancomycin to be administered intravenously for a week as well. A nurse is not allowed to administer intravenous antibiotics without a prescription. So, the intravenous antibiotics will be initiated after the prescription has been obtained. The patient might be put on Vancomycin 1 g daily or 1 g twice daily taking into consideration the renal function of the patient. If the patient has some renal dysfunction, the nephrologist will be involved to suggest and give guidance on an appropriate renal dose. Vancomycin is not combined with rifampicin as irrigations are not put on a patient with an implant. The Implants are removed before a DRI procedure is done on a patient. Microbiologists and Infectious Diseases physicians are also involved once a patient cultures and is started on antibiotics.

For a patient to be considered cleared of infection; they should have three consecutive negative culture results. If a patient has two negative specimen results and a third one is positive, the third one will cancel the first two negative ones and the patient will continue with irrigation treatment until they receive uninterrupted three negative specimen results.

6. Unblocking the irrigation system

At any given time, the irrigation system can be blocked. This can be observed during drainage times. When the yellow clip is opened there will be no movement of the fluid from the patient to the bellow. A bellow is supposed to provide a continuous negative suction pressure at all times but this would be disturbed due to various reasons. Those reasons might be after physiotherapy, after mobilizing to the bathroom without taking precaution in the handling of irrigation system or a blood cloth or fat debris from the bone marrow caught between the outside tube (the tube that drains the irrigation fluid from the patient) and the intra-catheter (the inner tube that administers antibiotic to the wound site).

Before trying to unblock the tubes, the system should be checked if it is still in situ, as the system is only held by one stitch around the insertion area, it is easy for tubes to come out. Once the tubes are out, the whole system must be removed. They must never be pushed back inside the patient as this is a sterile procedure done in theater, so pushing the irrigation system in the patient's wound would be introducing infection to the patient as those tubes would already have been exposed to the unsterile environment.

Another thing that a nurse can do to maintain the continuous negative suction is to open a blue or white clip between the bellow and a drain bag (That looks like a urine bag but without the volume markings) and then put pressure on the bellow until all the contents of the bellow have been drained to the drain bag. If the drain bag is full of air from the bellow, the air can be released without contaminating the system. If the bag is full of fluid drainage it can be emptied and discarded. There is no need to measure the contents of the bag.

If putting pressure on the bellow is not working a 20 ml syringe can be used as the same procedure of taking a specimen to try and provide manual suction. This can be done several times if the patient is complaining of pain. The clot; unless it is not big might come and may be seen in the syringe after being caught. The port must be closed and then the two pinch clamps (the red and yellow one) must be open to check if there is any drainage. If the clot was properly removed, the system might be seen running properly at this moment.

If those two avenues have been exhausted it could mean there is a clot somewhere that could not be removed with a mere 20 *ml* syringe. A 50 mg of Actilyse (alteplase) should be mixed with 50 ml of sterile water for injections. After that 2 *ml* of that solution should be added to an already prepared new solution of 50 *ml* sodium chloride and a relevant antibiotic. The 2 ml of alteplase solution should not be added to an already running antibiotic. A new solution must be prepared and an old one must be discarded so that 2 mg of actilyse is added into 50 ml of sodium chloride with for example 1.2 g of Augmentin.

Streptokinase 1,500,000 international units is another drug of choice in the unblocking of irrigation systems depending on the hospital pharmacy availability. It also should be added in 50 ml water for injection and 2 ml withdrawn and added into the antibiotics.

Two cycles of irrigation procedure should be enough to clear any clot and the solution should be removed unless the problem is persistent. The patient should also be monitored for any bleeding on the wound site. The solution should be discontinued if the bleeding is concerning or if it is disproportionate to the amount of antibiotic solution administered.

Sometimes the irrigation system will stop running and restart during the next cycle on its own without any interference from the nursing staff. The assumption is that there might be nothing to drain from inside especially after taking a specimen. Remember +/− 40 ml is taken during specimen collection and during the administration of antibiotics only 20 drops are administered, which is not a lot by any account.

7. Discussion

Patients are discouraged from mobilizing unnecessary to prevent pulling out of irrigation tubes. If a patient wants to go to the bathroom a plastic bag can be used to put the tubes, bellow, and drain bag in and the patient can carry it with the hand that is on the side of the limb with irrigations, for example, if the irrigations are on the left leg, the plastic bag should be carried on the left hand. The irrigation system should not be made to move across to the other side.

The patient is encouraged to reduce smoking; though this is a difficult thing to do the patient should be made aware that smoking will delay the process of wound healing [5].

If possible; the patient should not sleep on his own pajamas or blankets. They should use hospital linen, which can be changed daily so that the patient is nursed on a clean environment at all times. As the world has been engulfed by COVID-19 pandemic, most hospitals have changed their rules as far as visiting relatives are concerned, so it might be impossible for the family to bring clean pajamas every day for their relatives. The patient is also encouraged to take high protein foods to promote wound healing.

Author details

Princess Busisiwe Siphiwe Mbatha
Charlotte Maxeke Johannesburg Academic Hospital, Department of Orthopedics, Johannesburg, South Africa

*Address all correspondence to: bathaphiwe@gmail.com

References

[1] Blom A, Warwick D, Whitehouse M. Apley and Solomon's System of Orthopaedics and Trauma. 2018. pp. 31-43

[2] The Management of Chronic Osteomyelitis using Lautenbach Method [Internet]. National Library of Medicine. Bethesda; 2004. Available from: http://www.pubmed.ncbi.nlmnih.gov [Cited: 11 December 2021]

[3] Modified Lautenbach Technique in the Treatment of an Open Infected Non-union of the Clavicle—A Case Report [Internet]. Acta Orthopaedica. United Kingdom: Nordic Orthopaedic Federation; 2012. Available from: http://www.ncbi.nlm.nih.gov [Cited: 17 November 2021]

[4] Local Antibiotic Instillation and Suction Drainage after Surgery for Bone & Soft Tissue Infection [Internet]. South Africa; 2006. Available from: http://www.boneinfection.co.za/Irrigation_HandOut_v107.pdf [Cited: 10 December 2021]

[5] Smoking Greatly Increases Risk of Complications after Surgery [Internet]. Switzerland: WHO; 2020. Available from: https://www.who.int/news/item [Cited: 12 December 2021]

Chapter 9

STARZ-DRP: An Advance Nursing Approach for Palliative Home Care Services

Nazri Nordin

Abstract

Nurses perform a significant role as professional practitioners in the healthcare system, particularly providing the Palliative Home Care Services (PHCS). PHCS is a continuum of medical and social services which support the needs of patients living with chronic medical conditions or severe disabilities. Most of the time, they shall engage with patients and their family members in the absence of physicians or pharmacists. They shall assist them to go through their daily routines with physical help and support. Foremost, they shall help their patients to consume medications as being prescribed. For that reason, they need an advanced approach to assist them to provide a quality and excellent PHCS. Therefore, this article shall highlight a tool is known as STARZ-DRP as a potential modus operandi to maneuver them to make an accurate and quick triaging-decision as well as identify the actual or potential drug-related problems. It is to be hoped that the tool shall enhance the image of nurses as healthcare providers.

Keywords: palliative home care services, nurses, STARZ-DRP, pharmaceutical care, triaging-decision, drug-related problems

1. Introduction

Nursing practice is a critical profession in the healthcare system. Nurses are trained with a particular skill or type of behavior through practice and instruction over a period of time to assist the physicians in many aspects of tasks. Their ultimate role has the intention to reduce the burden of work of the physicians. They shall help the physicians to administer medicines, monitor desired or undesired medical conditions as well as provide sufficient or essential health welfare. Such a course of action acquires the nurses to learn or develop a particular skill, habit, or quality as a way to reflect their image as competent healthcare worker. Therefore, they must gain or acquire knowledge of or skill in a particular task by study, experience, or being formally taught. The process of learning shall maneuver them to integrate the essential knowledge, skills, perception, and behavior into their actual activities [1]. Sometimes, they must take the challenge to move forward from their comfortable way of practice towards more advanced knowledge and skills [2]. It shall benefit them and enhance their image in the healthcare system.

Nurses are having the chance to provide and lead a Palliative Home Care Service (PHCS) as a way to optimize quality of life and mitigate suffering among people with serious and complex illnesses [3]. Their roles in PHCS are well notified in many scientific writing papers [4]. Nonetheless, Sekse et al. noticed that they need additional knowledge and training, guidance, and support to fulfill their role in PHCS [4]. It is because the nurses might have to be in the state of being independent. PHCS is patient and family-centered care that optimizes quality of life by decreasing the suffering of continuum illnesses [3]. Most of the time, the patients might stay at home instead of the hospital. Such a scenario might reflect the absence of regular physician's attendance or attention. As a result, the nurses should take the responsibility to be key decision maker in the PHCS [5]. To ensure the high standard provision of tailored PHCS to patients with life-threatening illnesses and their relatives, the nurses need all their knowledge of basic nursing with additional and adequate skills. Such knowledge and skills might have the chance to make the nurses ready to deal with the challenges in term of practice, relationship with the patient and family members, and their self-motivation. Furthermore, the PHCS always demands on their role to be in a comprehensive way.

Among the essential knowledge and skills acquired in the PHCS are making a quick and accurate triaging decision [6]. Such a role needs the nurses to perceive the significance, explanation, or cause of triaging action. They must be knowledgeably aware of the character or nature of their patient's medical condition, particularly the illnesses which acquire immediate medical attention or examination. In addition to that, they must have the skills to identify, prevent, and resolve the actual or potential drug-related problems (DRP) [7]. Moreover, they should aware of their patient's drug-related needs [8]. The entire mode of action might have the chance to protect their patients from harm and danger of medication use and undesired diseases or condition.

This article shall highlight a potential approach is known as STARZ-DRP to maneuver the nurses to provide an efficient and competent PHCS [9]. STARZ-DRP had demonstrated its ability, capability, competence, and quality to make an accurate and quick triaging decision as well as identify, prevent, and resolve DRPs [10]. Foremost, the tool shall have the chance to assist the nurses to response to their patients' drug-related needs [10]. Therefore, STARZ-DRP had been acknowledged its values as a potential approach to give professional help and advice to patients in the healthcare system [11]. It is to be hoped that the approach shall enhance the importance, worth, or usefulness of PHCS in eyes of patients, their family members, policymakers, and other healthcare providers.

2. STARZ-DRP

2.1 Essential behavior

Nurses who provide PHCS must act or conduct themselves appropriately in response to a particular situation or practice. Such attitudes ensure they have a desire to perform the exact duties or services. Firstly, they must be ready to engage in providing PHCS. PHCS is constantly carried out at the place where the patient lives permanently. For such scenario, they must also possess the skills to communicate effectively or be involved directly with a member of their patient's family [12]. Otherwise, the family members might not have the chance to be actively interested in and concerned for the success of PHCS. Furthermore, the patient needs for assistance especially financial support as necessities for PHCS.

In addition to that, they must have considerable skills to communicate with the necessary confidentiality with other healthcare providers [13]. They should share or exchange information, news, or ideas using the principal method of communication which consists of comprehensive words in a structured and conventional mode and conveyed by speech, writing, or gesture [13]. Such communication skills should include or deal with all or nearly all elements or aspects of PHCS. The elements shall ensure the successful conveying or sharing of ideas and feelings by speaking, writing, or using some other mediums. Foremost, it shall make PHCS recognized, familiar, or within the scope of knowledge of patients and other healthcare providers.

They should have the ability to understand and share the feelings of another, particularly with the patients or their family members. Nonetheless, the feelings should be emphasized in the context of empathy. Such course of action shall ensure their feelings are not being bonded with their patients or family members. Moudatsou et al. notified that healthcare providers with high levels of empathy are having the chance to elicit better therapeutic outcomes [14]. The empathetic relationship between nurse and patient shall reinforce the need to complete the drug therapy plan as a way to achieve a desired outcome in the absence of medical or medication errors [15]. As a consequence, it shall enhance the quality of PHCS.

2.2 STARZ-DRP: a tool to provide a PHCS

STARZ-DRP is a simple mnemonic which established to assist the healthcare providers to make an accurate triage-decision as well as identify, prevent, and resolve the actual or potential drug-related problem. STARZ-DRP was developed by a group of clinical researchers from Universiti Sains Malaysia, Malaysia to meet a specified degree which proposed by the philosophy of Pharmaceutical Care (PC) [9]. The philosophy of PC acquires the healthcare providers to response to the patients' drug-related needs [16]. In addition to that, PC maneuvers them to identify, prevent, and resolve the actual or potential drug-related problems (DRPs) [16]. Such course of action is critical to put in the picture because DRPs shall have the chance to cause someone to be vulnerable or at risk of death or decrease his or her health quality of life. Whereas, an act of reacting quickly or positively to drug-related needs of an individual shall persuade the patient to meet the aims of PHCS as well as enhance compliance behavior towards therapy plan.

STARZ-DRP had involved in the previous study to determine its feasibilities to perform an accurate and quick triaging action as well as exercise a particular ability to proficiency identify, prevent, and resolve DRPs repeatedly or regularly [10]. Foremost, each component in STARZ-DRP was evaluated and estimated by a group of physicians and pharmacists to ascertain its nature, ability, and quality of making a triage-decision and identify the actual or potential DRPs [17]. Therefore, STARZ-DRP is having a chance to maneuver the healthcare provider to be an expert with adequate skill and knowledge in a particular field.

STARZ-DRP (**Table 1**) consists of the five most significantly original and influential alphabetic characters (S-T-A-R-Z). The first letter, **S**, represents the patient's presenting symptoms. The second letter, **T**, denotes the time of onset and duration of the presenting symptoms. The third letter, **A**, stands for the associated or related symptoms. The fourth letter, **R**, stands for recurrence or repeated symptoms. 'S-T-A-R' shall maneuver the nurses to evaluate or estimate the nature of patients' complaints about medical or medication issues. 'S-T-A-R' consists of specific questions, particularly in an official context as reflected in **Table 1**. Lastly, 'Z' means zoom into the patient's medical and

Alphabetical character	Description
S	Symptom presentation refers to subjective evidence of health problem perceived by the patient.
T	Time of onset and duration of the present symptoms.
A	Associated symptoms refer to patient symptoms explored and determined by the nurse during the interview. It does not refer to the symptoms presented earlier by the patient. This is done by using the pictorial documentation form. To aid and ease the nurse during the interview, the human body is arbitrarily divided into four regions: (1) Front: the part of the body facing the nurse (asking for symptoms like bloating, heartburn, nausea, vomiting, breathlessness, extra), (2) Back (asking for symptoms like lower and upper back pain, shoulder pain, and neck pain), (3) Upper (head) (asking for symptoms like headache, dizziness, problems with sleep, extra), and (4) Lower (asking for symptoms like numbness in both legs and hands, constipation, and swollen feet). Perhaps, the method is likened to a filtering or screening process to rule out the presence of severe symptoms.
R	Recurrence problem refers to the symptoms have been treated before, precisely when the symptoms recur and persist despite the treatment prescribed.
Z	Zoom into the patient's medication experience refers to information collected by the nurse related to any medical problems (for example, hypertension, diabetes, hyperthyroid, and extra), medication utilization (for example, use of prescription and non-prescription drugs, and herbal supplements), immunization history, allergies, drug sensitivities, drug side effects, adverse reactions, and the consumption of alcohol, caffeine, and tobacco.

[a]*This is not a diagnostic tool, rather it is a format with the purpose of organizing a nurse's knowledge in a manner that allows him/her to begin identifying the actual and potential DRPs and subsequently referring triage patients to the appropriate healthcare professionals.*
[b]*The patient's vital signs will be measured when necessary. At times, the patient's blood pressure, pulse rate, and body temperature are measured to aid the nurses in assessing the appropriateness of symptoms for self-medication.*

Table 1.
Definition of alphabetical characters in STARZ[a, b].

medication experience. Carefully guides the nurses to assess and evaluate medical and medication histories. 'Z' encourages them to devote their theoretical and practical understanding of clinical knowledge and experience to determine if the medical condition needs either medication or medical attention (**Table 1**). Therefore, the entire modus operandi of STARZ-DRP must be accomplished successfully as a way to ensure they do not fail to notice, hear, understand and keep in writing essential or critical information. Otherwise, PHCS shall be the absence of degree of excellence, abilities, qualities, or achievements.

Role to determine DRPs is a vigorous action in PHCS [18]. Such activity shall ensure the safety of patients when they start to consume medications [18]. STARZ-DRP is able to maneuver the nurses to identify a wide range of DRPs as notified in **Table 2**. Nonetheless, they should have adequate knowledge of pharmacological of basic therapeutic as a way to enhance their skill to perform the activities. For that reason, they should attend an accredited training involving those experts who are very knowledgeable about or skillful in identifying, preventing, and resolving DRPs. Furthermore, the trainers shall be a source of information if they want to ascertain something.

Interestingly, STARZ-DRP is able to be used or obtained in a documentation form (see **Figure 1** – Pharmacy Self-care Advice Form) [19]. The form eases them to evaluate the nature of the patient's complaint, a physical or mental feature, medical condition, and medication histories [19]. Such documentation activities shall provide information or

Indication	DRP#1: No indication for non-prescription medicine DRP#2: Uncertainty about the indication of drug DRP#3: Need for additional therapy
Effectiveness	DRP#4: Inappropriate drug choice DRP#5: Dose too low DRP#6: Ineffective therapy DRP#7: Interference with medical therapy by smoking/alcohol consumption DRP#8: Lack of understanding of the medication DRP#9: Monitoring required
Safety	DRP#10: Use of medication to which the patient is allergic DRP#11: Adverse drug events DRP#12: Potential drug-disease interaction DRP#13: Potential drug-drug interaction DRP#14: Dose too high
Compliance	DRP#15: Problems arising from the financial impact of therapy DRP#16: Interference with medical therapy by cultural/religious beliefs DRP#17: Failure of the patient to adhere to labelling instructions DRP#18: Others

Table 2.
List of DRPs.

evidence that serves as a permanent record for later reference. Furthermore, the course of action ensures the nurses might not fail to include critical information for further detailed examination. Foremost, the documentation form makes sure the nurse and patient have in or be able to bring to one's mind an awareness of something from the past.

Nurses shall have the chance to put in the picture their conclusion or resolution reached after considering the latter information in a documentation form as reflected in **Figure 1**. They shall write down their triaging decision if the patient needs a specific medication, referral for urgent medical attention, or further health screening test or examination. In addition to that, they shall draw special attention to DRPs by pointing out them in the form (**Figure 2**). Such documentation shall help them to evaluate and monitor the effectiveness of their essential actions.

Referral activities can be performed using a form that is reflected in **Figure 3**. The form shall have the chance to ease them to share or exchange critical information with other healthcare providers, particularly physicians and pharmacists. They can highlight the reason of referral as well as a category of DRPs to make physicians or pharmacists aware of a fact or circumstance. Subsequently, the other healthcare providers are able to take immediate action and behave in a specified way to resolve the medical problem. Such act of referral might have the chance to enhance the good quality and excellent of PHCS.

STARZ-DRP is having the chance to maneuver them to provide an excellent service in PHCS. A step-by-step approach notified in the modus operandi shall help them to make an accurate and quick triaging-decision as well as identify, prevent, and resolve DRPs. Foremost, the official documentation shall have the chance to establish a collaboration working relationship with other physician or pharmacist as a way to improve their patient's health quality of life.

2.3 Vital signs and symptoms

Nurses must be ready to methodically and systematically assess the essential information to evaluate and determine their patient's chief complaint. For that

Patient Name | Date

PHARMACY SELF-CARE ADVICE FORM

Demographic Information

I/C number : Gender : ☐ Male ☐ Female
Home Address :
Race : ☐ Malay ☐ Chinese ☐ Indian ☐ Other :
Religion : ☐ Muslim ☐ Christian ☐ Buddhist ☐ Hindu ☐ Other :
Marital status : ☐ Single ☐ Married
Occupation : ☐ Employee ☐ Self-Employed ☐ Unemployed ☐ Retired ☐ Housewife

Contact

Hse phone :
Cell-phone :
E-mail :

A. Request Related To : (check all that apply)

☐ Treatment for condition : | ☐ A specific product : | ☐ Other, specify :

(1). Check patients' signs and symptoms

1. State sign and symptom (refer figure 1.0) :
2. Duration :
3. Other associated symptom
   ☐ Yes (specify) :
   ☐ No
4. Recurrence sign and symptom
   ☐ Yes
   ☐ No

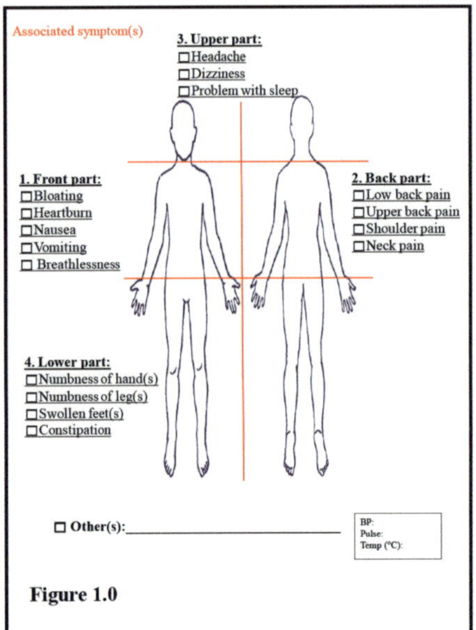

(2). Zoom to identify drug-related problem

1. Have you tried some products to resolve the problem ?
   ☐ Yes ☐ No
   Specify the product ::
2. Have you consulted a doctor to resolve the problem ?
   ☐ Yes ☐ No
   Specify the product :
3. Do you have a known medical problem ?
   ☐ Yes ☐ No
   Type of medical problem and how long :
4. Are you allergic to any drug or other substance ?
   ☐ Yes ☐ No
   Type of drug/substance :
5. Are you taking any prescription drug ?
   ☐ Yes ☐ No
   Specify the product :
6. Are you taking any other medications/herbals/supplements ?
   ☐ Yes ☐ No
   Specify the product :
7. Do you use of alcohol/caffeine/tobacco ?
   ☐ Yes ☐ No
   Specify the use:
8. Do you stop taking medication when you feel better ?
   ☐ Yes ☐ No
9. Do you stop taking medication when you feel worse ?
   ☐ Yes ☐ No
10. Do you have any concern about the cost of therapy ?
   ☐ Yes ☐ No
11. Are you pregnant ? (Optional question)
   ☐ Yes ☐ No

Figure 1.
Pharmacy self-care advice form.

reason, they must establish or indicate who or what are the critical signs and symptoms that acquire for immediate medical attention or examination. **Table 3** reflects the signs and symptoms that need intervention by the physicians [20].

Among signs and symptoms that are serious to handle themselves are abnormal readings of systolic and diastolic, heart rate, and body temperature (forehead,

(3). Sign and Symptom Assessment

The presenting signs/symptoms is/are NOT easily recognized as self-treatable condition ?	The presenting signs/symptoms is/are too serious for self-treatment ?	The patient requires further medical examination ?
☐ Yes ☐ No	☐ Yes ☐ No	☐ Yes ☐ No

(4). Pharmacy Care Plan

☐ Recommended	☐ Referral	☐ Health screening/promotion
Specify : ☐ OTC product ☐ Poison C & D ☐ Herbal product ☐ Homeopathic product ☐ Other, specify :	Specify : ☐ General practitioner (GP) ☐ Hospital ☐ Conditional referral to GP (if not better in # of days)	Specify : ☐ BP measurement ☐ Pregnancy test ☐ Blood cholesterol ☐ Blood/Urine glucose ☐ Other, specify :
List of product :	Reason for referral :	Describe advice :

(5). Follow-up

Provide reasons and how to :

B. States Drug-Related Problem

Indication	Effectiveness	Safety	Compliance
☐ No indication for non-prescription medication ☐ Uncertainty about the indication of drug ☐ Need for additional therapy	☐ Inappropriate drug choice ☐ Dose too low ☐ Ineffective therapy ☐ Interference with medical therapy by alcohol /caffeine/smoking consumption ☐ Lack of understanding of the medication ☐ Monitoring required	☐ Use of medication to which the patient is allergic ☐ Adverse drug events ☐ Potential drug –disease interaction ☐ Potential drug-drug interaction ☐ Dose too high	☐ Problems arising from financial impact of therapy ☐ Interference with medical therapy by cultural/religious beliefs ☐ Failure of the patient to adhere to labeling instructions ☐ Others

Figure 2.
Drug related problems.

tympanic, or rectal). In addition to that, too many associated symptoms, frequent emergence undesired symptoms, or too long-suffering of unresolved symptoms notified among the patients might reflect the actual or potential unexpected, undesired, untreated, or unresolved medical conditions. Foremost, it might suggest as potentially harmful or threatening to the patients' life. For such course of action, they should urgently contact or inform the physician or pharmacist as a way to resolve the condition.

Undesired or unresolved signs and symptoms should be and must be evaluated or estimated its natures if they need for a medication or a medication is the main cause.

To enhance communication between physician and pharmacist for the patient benefit.

PATIENT REFERRAL FORM

FROM:
Pharmacist:
Phone:
Address:

ATTENTION TO:
Doctor:
Phone:
Address:

Regarding Patient/Customer: I/C number:

I'm concerned about the following problems and wish to call it to your attention:

(i) Related to the patient's presenting signs/symptoms

(ii) Related to the patient's medication use

(iii) Related to the patient's factors:

I Recommend:

☐ Further assessment & examination

☐ Need additional therapy:

☐ Resolve the drug related problem

Please contact me as soon as possible, so we can provide the best care possible to the patient.

Thank You

Figure 3.
Patient referral form.

Such a particular condition requires the nurses to collaborate with the physician and pharmacist to determine an appropriate therapy plan. Their expert skill or knowledge in a particular field might have the chance to resolve the undesired medical condition.

1.	Any chest pain in a patient looking grey, sweating, or ill
2.	Severe pain in the chest, abdomen, head, or ears
3.	Blood loss from any orifice
4.	Increasing breathlessness
5.	Difficulty in swallowing
6.	Tenderness over blood vessels
7.	A history of severe injury, particularly a penetrating injury, or loss of consciousness
8.	Persistent raised temperature, blood pressure, or heart rate
9.	Loss of weight
10.	Anorexia
11.	Yellow skin colour
12.	Ankle swelling
13.	Yellow or green sputum
14.	Yellow or green discharge from penis or vagina
15.	Urinary symptoms
16.	Any menstrual abnormality
17.	Any swelling or lump of any size, including joints
18.	Weakness in arms or legs
19.	Any visual changes

Table 3.
Signs and symptoms that need urgent medical attention.

For example, the pharmacist might perform a therapeutic drug monitoring test as a potential approach to establish exactly an appropriate dose of a particular medication for an individual patient. The course of action shall ensure the patient is the absence of undesired adverse drug reactions. Foremost, an accurate dose of a medication shall provide an assurance that the patient might gain the benefits of such therapy.

2.4 Drug-related problems

Nurses must identify, prevent, and resolve the actual or potential DRPs among the patients who consume medications. Such a role shall have a chance to magnify the values of PHCS as well as have an effect on the character, development, or behavior of patients towards the service. For example, undesired side-effects or adverse drug reactions shall cause the patients to refuse to consume a specific medication. In addition to that, failure to resolve the medical condition might give rise to an idea that the patient might potentially dispose to agree with the medication's dosage regimen or its route of administration. For that reason, the nurses should have adequate training to ensure each medication is indicated, safe, and effective [21]. Foremost, they must ensure the patients are complying with the medication's dosage regimen [21].

Indicated: nurses must be ready to determine if the patients require an additional prescription or non-prescription medication to alleviate or resolve the illnesses or undesired and unexpected medical conditions. They must inform and advise the physician about the justification for the need of such medication. Such course of action shall make sure the medication is having the chance to eliminate disease or relieve them of undesired signs and symptoms.

Effectiveness: each medication must be effective to alleviate or resolve the unwanted medical condition. For that reason, they must collaborate with the physician to carefully choose medication as being the best or most suitable. Afterward, they should monitor and inform the physician about the effectiveness of the medication to resolve the medical problem. For example, they can appraise the physicians of the potential dose is too low for their patients. In addition to that, they should determine if there are other factors that interfere with medication intake to decrease its effectiveness. For example, the consumption of alcohol [22], caffeine [23], and smoking [24] are having the chance to interrupt the effectiveness of some medications. In other words, they can look at closely or with interest their patients on behalf of physicians about desired or undesired outcomes before or after consuming a specific medication.

Safety: all medications must not cause unwanted effects to the patients such as undesired side-effects or adverse drug reactions (ADRs). Undesired side-effects might have the potential to set or serve as a limit to the patients' daily activities. For example, the patient might feel too sleepy and hard to be awake the whole day after consuming a tablet of *Chlorpheniramine*. Whereas, ADRs might cause life-threatening if not immediately being treated. For example, there is a tendency for a gouty-patient to experience extremely ADRs such as *Stephen-Johnson Syndrome* after consuming a tablet of *Allopurinol*. For that reason, they must ensure each medication is the absence of potential allergic to the patient, ADRs, potential drug-disease or drug–drug interaction, as well as too high dose.

Compliance: the accomplishment of an aim or purpose of the therapy plan determined by the compliance behavior among the patients. Failure to comply with the dosage regimen might have a chance to make the medical condition become worse or even not being well treated. For that reason, they must identify the actual or potential factors which have an effect on the incompliance behavior. For example, the problem that arises from the financial impact of therapy or interference by cultural or religious beliefs might be the factors. Those factors can be eliminated if the patients are well educated about the critical needs of such a therapy plan. Therefore, the nurses must have adequate training as good educator.

2.5 Clinical parameters to monitor

They must also be aware of the facts, information, and skills acquired through experience or education the theoretical or practical understanding of laboratory-based health screening tests [25]. Such a test shall provide comprehensive information in revealing the degree to which the medical problems are in good health. In addition, it shall reflect the effectiveness of certain medications to alleviate or resolve a specific medical condition. For example, the hematology profile might have the chance to reflect the conditions of red blood cells and hemoglobin and their characters. Lack of both substances shall have an effect on the oxygen level in the bloodstreams. Whereas, the renal profile might give consideration to the selection of medications that have less undesired effects on the kidneys. The liver profile shall give a rise to awareness of medications that are potentially harmful to the liver. Lipid profile shall maneuver the practitioner to determine the effectiveness of statin drugs to lower the cholesterol readings. In short, the entire information obtained in the test shall have a chance to assist them towards an excellence way of performing PHCS in the healthcare system.

They should also work jointly with physicians on an activity to determine the effectiveness of the therapy plan through results such as *X-Ray* [26], *Magnetic Resonance Image* [27], or else. Such advanced medical technologies are helpful to give an exact topography of internal organs which reflect actual or potential abnormalities. Any findings obtained from the test shall maneuver them to be more focused on providing a specific therapy plan. In addition, it shall ensure the end result obtained from the test shall be the center of interest or activity.

Foremost, they should determine PHCS is able to enhance the health quality of life of their patients. They can utilize EQ-5D questionnaire as a tool to assess the clinical parameter [28]. The tool consists of two parts: (1). descriptive assessment which comprises of five domains—mobility, self-care, usual activities, pain or discomfort, and anxiety or depression, (2). visual analog scale to indicate the general health status with 100 indicating the best health status. Such a tool is easier to use and it is helpful while providing PHCS.

2.6 Barriers

A role to identify, prevent, and resolve DRPs is not well-known in nursing practice. Nonetheless, they should take the responsibility to perform such a role because it has had a chance to keep undesired ADRs from happening. ADRs are potentially life-threatening. For that reason, they must take the role of a medication protector in the absence of physicians and pharmacists. They are ready to take, hold, or deploy the skills to determine DRPs even though the basic training might consume cash and time respectively.

STARZ-DRP which has a chance to maneuver them to identify, prevent, and resolve DRPs was patented under the Copyright Act 1987 by Universiti Sains Malaysia with a reference number is CRLY00004047. It was ethically approved to perform towards patients in the previous studies by Universiti Sains Malaysia—Lam Wah Ee Hospital Joint Committee for Clinical Study Ethics (reference number is USM-HLWE/IEC/2008(0026) and Human Research Ethics Committee Universiti Sains Malaysia Centre for Research Initiatives, Clinical and Health Sciences, Universiti Sains Malaysia Health Campus (reference number is USM/JEPeM/15040145). For that reason, it is essential to officially inform the author if they would like to utilize STARZ-DRP as their modus operandi.

2.7 Perception to STARZ-DRP

STARZ-DRP is having constructive, optimism, or confidence among other healthcare providers such as physicians and pharmacists. Their responses had been published in other scientific journals [29]. For that reason, the approach might have the chance to establish an excellent working collaboration relationship with other healthcare providers. In addition, the experts in the healthcare system had notified STARZ-DRP as a potential approach to make an accurate and quick triaging decision as well as identify, prevent, and resolve the actual or potential DRPs. Foremost, the stakeholders noticed the potential of the approach to assess and counsel patients respectively [29].

3. Conclusion

STARZ-DRP is a potential approach for PHCS to enhance their skills to make a triaging decision and determine DRPs or the needs of their patients. Such course of action shall have the chance to enhance the excellent service of PHCS. Foremost, the approach shall assist them to ensure their patients are having the chance to improve their health quality of life.

Acknowledgements

Dr. Nazri Nordin is a Specialist in the field of Clinical Pharmacy who established the practice of Pharmaceutical Care in Malaysia through evidence-based clinical research while completing his Master of Science in Clinical Pharmacy and PhD in Clinical Pharmacy at Universiti Sains Malaysia, Malaysia. The module which is reflected via a simple mnemonic known as STARZ was patented under the Copyright Act 1987 by Universiti Sains Malaysia (Ref Num: CRLY00004047). It was approved to perform towards patients in the previous studies by Univesiti Sains Malaysia-Lam Wah Ee Hospital Joint Committee for Clinical Study Ethics (Ref Num:USM-HLWE/IEC/2008(0026) and Human Research Ethics Committee Universiti Sains Malaysia, Centre for Research Initiatives, Clinical & Health Sciences, Universiti Sains Malaysia Health Campus (Ref Num: USM/JEPeM/15040145).

Author details

Nazri Nordin
Universiti Sains Malaysia, Malaysia

*Address all correspondence to: drnazrinordin@gmail.com

References

[1] Takase M, Teraoka S, Miyakoshi Y, Kawada A. A concept analysis of nursing competence: A review of international literature. Nihon Kango Kenkyu Gakkai Zasshi. 2011;**34**:103-109

[2] Fukada M. Nursing competency: Definition, structure and development. Yonago Acta Medica. 2018;**61**(1):1-7. DOI: 10.33160/yam.2018.03.001

[3] Hagan TL, Xu J, Lopez RP, Bressler T. Nursing's role in leading palliative care: A call to action. Nurse Education Today. 2018;**61**:216-219. DOI: 10.1016/j.nedt.2017.11.037

[4] Sekse RJT, Hunskar I, Ellingsen S. The nurse's role in palliative care: A qualitative meta-synthesis. Journal of Clinical Nursing. 2018;**27**(1-2):e21-e38. DOI: 10.1111/jocn.13912

[5] Thompson C, Cullum N, McCaughan D, et al. Nurses, information use, and clinical decision making—The real world potential for evidence-based decisions in nursing. Evidence-Based Nursing. 2004;7:68-72

[6] Borasioa GD, Gamondib C, Obristc M, Joxd R. COVID-19: Decision making and palliative care. Swiss Medical Weekly. 2020;**150**:w20233

[7] Rémi C, Bauer D, Krumm L, Bausewein C. Drug-related problems on a palliative care unit. Journal of Pain & Palliative Care Pharmacotherapy. 2021;**2021**:1-9

[8] Al-Quteimat OM, Amer AM. Evidence-based pharmaceutical care: The next chapter in pharmacy practice. Saudi Pharmaceutical Journal. 2016;**24**(4):447-451. DOI: 10.1016/j.jsps.2014.07.010

[9] Sarriff A, Nordin N, Hassali MA. STARZ-DRP: A step-by-step approach for pharmacy triage services. Malaysia Journal of Pharmacy. 2011;**1**(9):311-326

[10] Nordin N, Sarriff A, Hassali MA. STARZ-DRP: A tool for pharmacy triage services. Asian Journal of Pharmaceutical and Clinical Research. 2017;**10**(10):151-157

[11] Taylor J, Rocchi M. The art and science of counselling patients on minor ailments/OTC medicines. SelfCare. 2018;**9**(3):3-22

[12] Kourkouta L, Papathanasiou IV. Communication in nursing practice. Mater Sociomed. 2014;**26**(1):65-67. DOI: 10.5455/msm.2014.26.65-67

[13] Maureen Nokuthula Sibiya. Effective Communication in Nursing, Nursing, Nilgun Ulutasdemir. IntechOpen; 2018. pp. 20-23 DOI: 10.5772/intechopen.74995

[14] Moudatsou M, Stavropoulou A, Philalithis A, Koukouli S. The role of empathy in health and social care professionals. Healthcare (Basel). 2020;**8**(1):26. DOI: 10.3390/healthcare8010026

[15] Hojat M, Louis DZ, Maio V, et al. Empathy and health care quality. American Journal of Medical Quality. 2013;**28**:6-7. DOI: 10.1177/1062860612464731

[16] Cipolle RJ, Strand LM, Morley PC. Pharmaceutical Care Practice: The Clinician's Guide. 2nd ed. New York: McGraw Hill; 2004

[17] Nordin N. A Qualitative and Quantitative assessment of STARZ-DRP for triage action plan, determine drug-related problems and counsel self-care

customers in Malaysia community pharmacies. Universiti Sains Malaysia (PhD). 2018

[18] Ellenbecker CH, Samia L, Cushman MJ, et al. Patient safety and quality in Home Health Care. In: Hughes RG, editor. Patient Safety and Quality: An Evidence-Based Handbook for Nurses. Rockville (MD): Agency for Healthcare Research and Quality (US); 2008

[19] Nordin N, Hassali MA. STARZ-DRP: Improving Efficiency of Patient Care in Community Pharmacies. InTechOpen 2020. DOI: 10.5772/intechopen.86021

[20] Holland R. When to Refer. Pharmaceutical Society of Australia. 1993. p. 15

[21] Hughes RG, Blegen MA. Medication administration safety. In: Hughes RG, editor. Patient Safety and Quality: An Evidence-Based Handbook for Nurses. Rockville (MD): Agency for Healthcare Research and Quality (US); 2008. Chapter 37. PMID: 21328757

[22] Weathermon R, Crabb DW. Alcohol and medication interactions. Alcohol Research Health. 1999;**23**(1):40-54

[23] Belayneh A, Molla F. The effect of coffee on pharmacokinetic properties of drugs: A review. BioMed Research International. 2020;**2020**:7909703. DOI: 10.1155/2020/7909703

[24] Kroon LA. Drug interactions with smoking. American Journal of Health-System Pharmacy. 2007;**64**(18): 1917-1921. DOI: 10.2146/ajhp060414

[25] Kee JL, Hayes ER. Assessment of patient laboratory data in the acutely ill. The Nursing Clinics of North America. 1990;**25**(4):751-759

[26] Myatt R. X-rays: What the nurse needs to know. Nursing Standard. 2017;**32**(1): 39-43. DOI: 10.7748/ns.2017.e10749

[27] Lima MS, Shigueoka DC, Salvador ME, et al. Assessment of nurses' knowledge about magnetic resonance imaging in a university hospital in Sao Paulo. International Journal of Nursing Practice. 2012 Dec;**18**(6):574-581. DOI: 10.1111/ijn.12011

[28] EuroQol Group. 30. EuroQol: A new facility for the measurement of health-related quality of life. Health Policy. 1990;**16**:199-208

[29] Nordin N, Hassali MA, Sarriff A. STARZ-DRP as a triaging tool for community pharmacists: Perspectives and expectations of stakeholders. International Journal of Pharmacy and Pharmaceutical Sciences. 2017;**9**(11):81-86